TMJ: ITS MANY FACES

Diagnosis of TMJ and Related Disorders

Second Edition

Wesley E. Shankland, II, D.D.S., Ph.D.

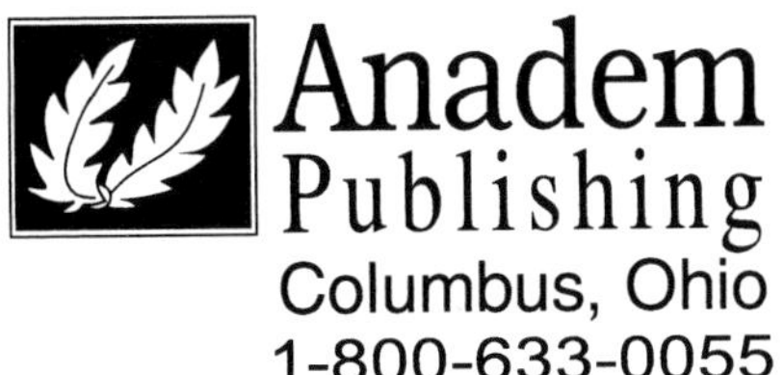

Columbus, Ohio
1-800-633-0055

TMJ: ITS MANY FACES
Diagnosis of TMJ And Related Disorders

Second Edition

Anadem Publishing, Inc.
Columbus, Ohio 43214
614•262•2539
800•633•0055

The material in *TMJ: Its Many Faces. Diagnosis of TMJ And Related Disorders, second edition* is presented for informational purposes only and it is not meant to be, and should not be relied upon for, recommendations regarding diagnosis or treatment for any individual case. It is not meant to be a substitute for proper medical care by your doctor. You need to consult with your doctor for diagnosis and treatment.

Dedication

This book is dedicated to all of those wonderful patients that I have had the privilege to know over the past 17 years who have suffered so much from a TMJ problem. They have taught me much about pain, suffering, and the human character.

This book is also dedicated to my lovely and wonderful wife, Cathy. She has been so patient with me over the past 26 years as I have pursued what I perceived as my calling. Her honesty, integrity, and humility are beyond reproach. What an example to our children and to me. I am eternally grateful for her partnership in my life. "Her children arise up and call her blessed; her husband also, and he praiseth her." (Proverbs 31:28)

I also wish to dedicate this book to my children: Wes, David and Carrie. They have been extremely understanding as Dad has gone back to school, kept his nose in books, written papers, and traveled far too much to lecture. Their forgiveness and support have been far greater than I deserve. They are hardly impressed with their father; good for them!

Lastly, and most importantly, this book is dedicated to my Savior and Lord, Jesus Christ. Taking me to this point, He is the reason that I have devoted my life to this present rewarding, yet challenging work.

Foreword

When I first met Dr. Wes Shankland in August 1991, I was suffering the worst pain of my life and no one could help me, despite the best efforts of some fine doctors. I didn't trust Dr. Shankland or his treatment at first, partly because I'd been disappointed so often in the past. Also, my cure was not instant, and who among us doesn't want immediate relief from pain?

Dr. Shankland had both faith in his treatment and persistence in encouraging me to stick with it, and eventually I was given complete recovery. I still have brief episodes of pain from time to time and given my personality, I don't always handle these recurrences well. But under Dr. Shankland's guidance and care, I have a normal, almost pain-free existence.

I firmly believe in his professional medical judgment, honed by many years of treating diverse kinds of pain, and in his sincere desire to help people who suffer chronic pain. I can testify that the hard splints he uses work. I've gained more long-term relief and **hope** from the splints he's made for me than from any other treatment, including surgery.

If you suffer from undiagnosed pain or if you think you might suffer from TMJ or TMJ-related pain, read this book carefully. It might do for you what it did for me: give you a new lease on life.

Jim Downard

February 1995

Acknowledgments

While a dental student at The Ohio State University, I studied with a very demanding professor, Dr. Richard Huffman. He demanded the best at all times; he would never compromise even when I felt that he should. I wish to thank him for the fine example and for discipling me.

In 1982, I met Dr. Edwin Ernest of Montgomery, Alabama. He was the most knowledgeable person concerning TMJ and associated disorders that I have yet to meet. Ed became my friend and my mentor. I owe much to him for his constant patience with me.

I'd like to thank my office staff: Cheryl McCutcheon, Pat Masucci, Kay Gentry, Jan Klepser, Bev Cholley, RN, and Karen Gallaugher, RDH. They are perhaps my biggest supporters and all tremendous women in the Lord. They pray for me, lift me up, and along with my wife, are my "self-appointed" humility enforcers. Thanks, ladies!

Thanks to Molly Klepser Denison for lending beauty to the back cover.

I also want to thank Sherry Messick for her inspiration; she showed me how essential it is for affected patients to have information about scleroderma and the TMJs.

I wish to thank my in-laws, David and Geneva Culp, for caring and lovingme and providing such a wonderful example of a loving couple. Happy 63rd this year!

Special thanks to the future Dr. Steve Fleshman for his advice and assistance with Chapter 13. The world will be a much better place when he finishes his Naturopathic Doctor degree.

Last but not least, I would like to thank my wonderful mother, Lorna Shankland. She has always been my greatest supporter. Her encouragement has meant more than she will ever know. Thanks Mom! (I really mean it!)

Table of Contents

Figures

Miscellaneous

Tables

Introduction

Billions of dollars are spent annually for many doctor, clinic, hospital, or therapist visits. Pain sufferers will do and pay anything for some hope of relief. Doctors either don't understand or believe them; family members (especially spouses) think nothing must be wrong because the learned doctors can find no explanations for the pain. It must be *stress*; or, it must be *all in their head*.

Have you heard these excuses before? If you are a typical TMJ sufferer, you probably have. Don't blame family members. They must rely on doctors' opinions. Doctors rely on what they have been taught. The poor soul suffering feels abandoned, left alone, misunderstood. He or she tries to cope, but sometimes the suffering seems unbearable, private, and many are brought to the brink of suicide. Some, sadly, step over the brink.

Head, facial, neck and even ear pain have many different causes. However, a dislocated temporomandibular joint (TMJ) or injury to many of the associated TMJ structures account for a very high percentage of pain in the head. If you have seen, as most of these unfortunate patients do, physicians, neurologists, otolaryngologists (ENT doctors), or even psychologists and no definite diagnosis has been made and no effective treatment has been recommended, then chances are you may be suffering from a TMJ problem.

For over 17 years I have practiced dentistry, with my primary efforts being directed toward the diagnosis and treatment of TMJ and related pain. Tremendous advances have been made in almost all areas of dentistry and medicine concerning pain management. However, the most important problem with TMJ treatment is that it's been ignored by many researchers. Why? Perhaps those in the research labs have never suffered or have not been married to a TMJ sufferer.

In 1983, we conducted a survey of our TMJ patients. We were not surprised to discover that our office was the 6th, on average, visited by TMJ sufferers. One patient had seen 19 previous doctors! Since then, I've seen one poor woman who had been to 31 other offices before making ours number 32. The two common denominators with these patients were:

1. The doctors apparently did not listen to the patients about their symptoms; or,

2. The doctors did not recognize a TMJ problem.

I will never say that our office correctly diagnoses and successfully treats every patient. That would be arrogant and unrealistic. I will say that in all my years of practice, I can only recall two or three patients who had a psychological problem producing their pain.

This book is not the final word on TMJ. Many other fine books have been written and some are listed in the reference section in the Appendix B. Further, the TMJ sufferer must realize that he or she has to play a big part in determining the proper diagnosis and subsequent treatment. Often, exercises, dietary improvements, or alterations in life-style may be all that need change. Sometimes the proper health care professional must be consulted. Some organizations of such practitioners are listed in the Appendix A. But remember, the sufferer must be actively involved in his or her treatment. Not only is it unrealistic, but also unfair, to rely only upon the doctor or therapist. They should be viewed as partners or guides. The patient is responsible for recovery, not the doctors.

As you read the following pages, remember that everyone is an individual and responds differently to the same type of treatment. Also, perhaps more than one type of treatment may be necessary in order to help your TMJ problem. Your body is far more complex than any computer or machine. In other words, we are "...fearfully and wonderfully made." (Psalm 139:14)

Just as James Downard has written in the preface of this book, there is hope for those who suffer with TMJ. Treatment is not always easy nor is there *ever* a promise of a total cure.

One

What Is TMJ?

Many people, even doctors, nurses, and insurance companies, use the term *TMJ*. But what does this abbreviation mean?

TMJ is an abbreviation for *temporomandibular joint*, or the jaw joint. There are two, one in front of each ear. The TMJ is the joint formed by the temporal bone of the skull (*temporo*) with the lower jaw or mandible (*mandibular*). Figure 1 shows the relationship of

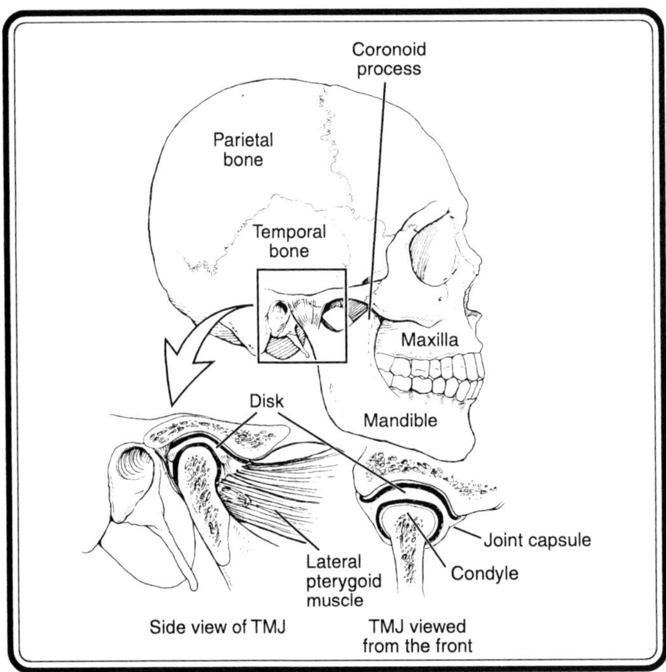

Figure 1: Anatomy of the TMJ

these bones as they form the temporomandibular joint. These joints move each time we chew, talk or swallow. They are probably the most used joints in the body (used far more by some of us than others!).

Today we know that TMJ is really a group of several disorders that usually have similar symptoms.

To accommodate this frequent use and to help us open our mouths wide, the TMJ is actually a sliding joint, not a ball-and-socket like the shoulder. This sliding allows for pressures placed on the joint to be distributed throughout the joint and not just in one area.

In the medical community, the term TMJ is really not correct. It designates an anatomical structure (the joint) and not a painful condition. The correct term, as recommended by the American Dental Association, is ***TMD,*** or *Temporomandibular Disorders*, a more precise term than TMJ. However, in this book TMJ will be used because it is so well known. So when we say *TMJ*, let's agree that we are talking about a condition that is often quite painful, debilitating, and frustrating.

But what is the condition of TMJ? In the strictest sense, TMJ is a set of separate and yet related disorders of the temporomandibular joints and associated structures. These structures include muscles, ligaments, tendons, nerves and blood vessels.

We used to think that TMJ was just one problem. Today we know that TMJ is really a group of several disorders that usually have similar symptoms. That is one of the main reasons why so many people continue to suffer from a TMJ disorder even though they are being treated by honest, well-meaning practitioners.

TMJ Anatomy

The temporomandibular joint is the most complex joint in the human body. It is formed by the connection (called *articulation)* of the lower jaw (the mandible) with the upper jaw (the temporal bone), as shown in Figure 1. Between these two bones is a disc, just like the one between your back bones. This disc is primarily made of cartilage and in the TMJ acts like a third bone. Because it is attached to a muscle, the disc actually moves with certain movements of the TMJ.

The nerve to the TMJ is a branch of the trigeminal nerve (ever heard of *trigeminal neuralgia?*) For this reason, an injury to the TMJ may be confused with neuralgia of the trigeminal nerve.

The temporomandibular joint is the most complex joint in the human body.

This is important to know: one TMJ can't function without affecting the other one. Put another way, if one TMJ is injured, the other joint will usually become affected sometime in the future. This is true for knees and ankles as well. Injured ligaments rarely completely heal; and this is especially true of those associated with the TMJ. Some of these ligaments of the TMJ are extremely small. The forces placed upon them by chewing make it nearly impossible for proper healing.

The two bones of the TMJ are held together by a series of ligaments, any of which can be damaged, just like any other joint. A damaged TMJ ligament usually results in a dislocation of the disc, the lower jaw, or both. Also, the bones are connected by two main muscles: the temporalis and the masseter. Either of these muscles may be painful and produce pain in the TMJ or abnormal movement of the lower jaw.

Muscles associated with the TMJ

There are many muscles in the head, neck and face that are associated with the TMJs. In fact, virtually all muscles of the neck, back, throat and face either directly or indirectly affect the TMJs. The primary muscles are termed the *muscles of mastication* and include the left and right temporalis, lateral and medial pterygoids, and the masseters. These muscles are all controlled by branches of the third division of the trigeminal nerve.

The temporalis and masseter muscles close the jaw. They work like the biceps muscle of the arm, which draws the hand up and towards the body. Both the temporalis and masseter are powerful muscles, capable together of applying as much as 750 to 1000 pounds of pressure on the teeth. No wonder fillings and cracked teeth can fracture so easily! It's also amazing that the TMJs can withstand such constant forces over our lifetimes. Sometimes they can't.

Both the temporalis and masseter are powerful muscles, capable together of applying as much as 750 to 1000 pounds of pressure on the teeth. It's amazing that the TMJs can withstand such constant forces. Sometimes they can't.

All of these muscles of mastication are paired: there is one on the right side and one on the left. The temporalis (*temple muscle*) attaches the entire side of the skull to the lower jaw at a prominent structure termed the *coronoid process* of the mandible (Figure 2). This powerful muscle closes the mouth and draws the jaw backwards, helping us to chew efficiently. Locate this muscle by lightly pushing against your temple and then clenching your teeth. Feel the slight bulge? That is the *anterior belly* of the temporalis. When the TMJ is injured or dislocated, it frequently is painful, kind of like a tension headache.

The masseter, too, is a powerful muscle and actually gets larger, just like the biceps, if someone clenches or grinds his or her teeth a lot. In concert with the temporalis muscles, the masseter muscles (one on each side) close the lower jaw and aid in chewing (Figure 3).

Lightly press your fingers against the sides of your face just below your cheeks and clench your teeth. Do

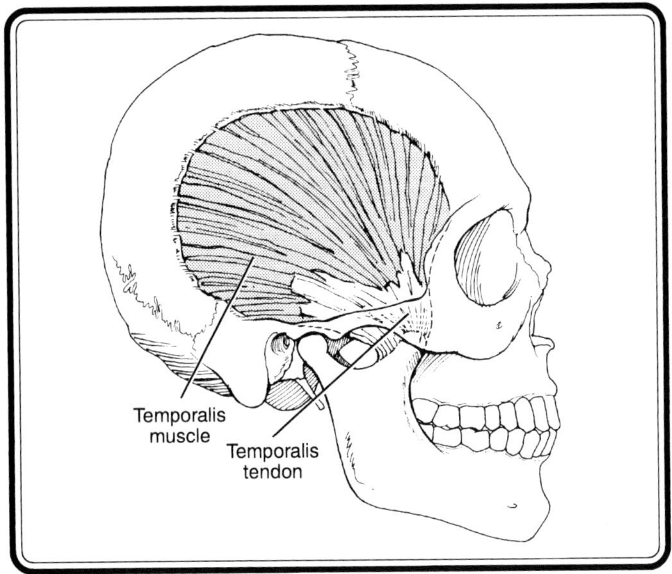

Figure 2: The temporalis muscle

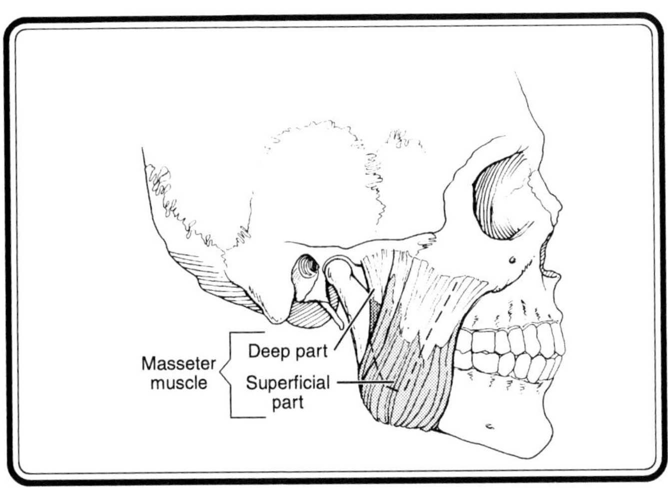

Figure 3: The masseter muscle

you feel the masseters bulge? Often, the masseters become sore after clenching, grinding, or an injury to the TMJ. Also, like the temporalis muscles, the masseters can enlarge when overused.

The lateral pterygoid muscles are similar to the temporalis and masseter and yet, quite different. The lateral pterygoid is composed of two portions or bellies, the superior and inferior (Figure 4).

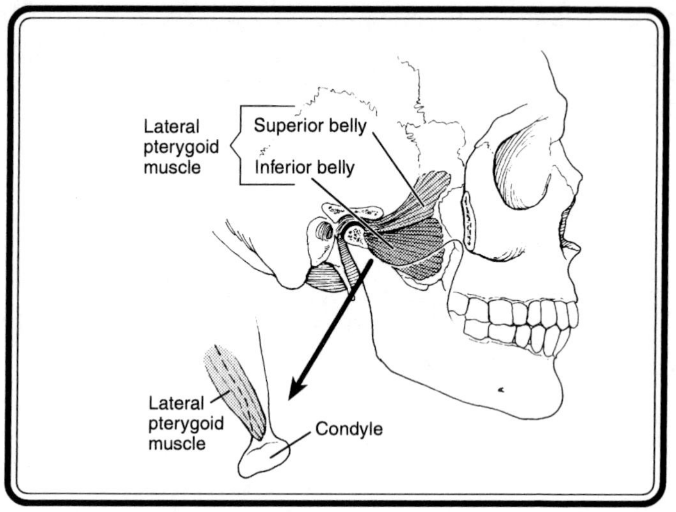

Figure 4: The lateral pterygoid muscle

The superior belly is primarily attached to the TMJ's articular disc and is responsible for proper disc movement in coordination with movement of the lower jaw, especially when closing the mouth.

By contrast, the inferior belly is predominately attached to the top of the lower jaw (the *mandibular condyle*) and is accountable for moving the lower jaw forward, thus opening the mouth, and pulling the mandible to one side. This belly works with muscles, known as *accessory muscles*, located in the throat just under the chin (primarily the mylohyoid, anterior digastric muscles) to open the mouth.

Even though the lateral pterygoid bellies work almost in opposition to each other, the same branch of the trigeminal nerve goes to both. Dislocation of the TMJ disc increases muscle tension in both, but especially the superior belly. This increased muscle tension can cause pain in the TMJ, the face, the maxillary sinus, or in and behind the eye. Consequently, if your disc is out of place, you may visit an eye doctor or ear, nose and throat specialist for eye or sinus pain when actually your pain is produced as a result of a displaced TMJ disc.

The fourth muscle of mastication, the medial pterygoid, assists the temporalis and masseter muscles in closing the mouth. This and the masseter muscle form a sling around the back end of the mandible (Figure 5). It runs parallel with the masseter but inside the jaw. Injury to this muscle produces pain in the TMJ, deep in the side of the head, the ear and even the maxillary sinus.

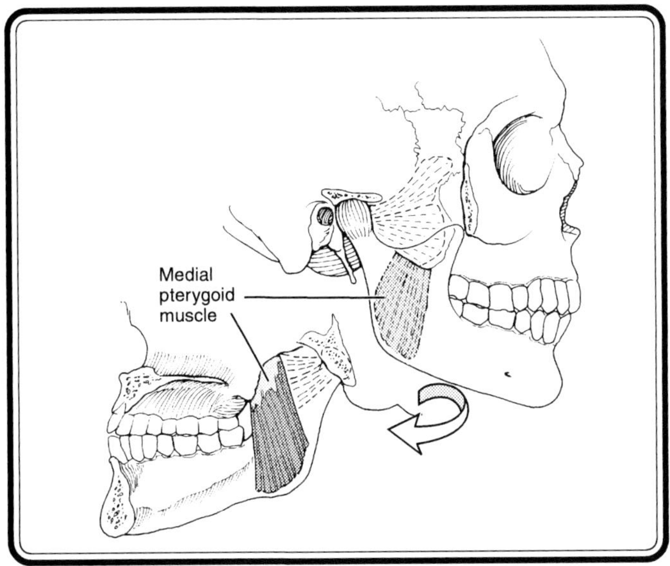

Figure 5: The medial pterygoid muscle

Neck muscles associated with the TMJ

The skull and mandible are precariously balanced on the spinal column by a complex series of muscles and the spinal column on the pelvis, also by an extensive series of muscles and ligaments. The entire upper body is in turn supported by the legs and ultimately the feet. Guess what? This lower body support is also by way of muscles.

Dislocation of the TMJ disc increases muscle tension in both bellies of the lateral pterygoid muscle. This increased muscle tension can cause pain in the TMJ, the face, the maxillary sinus, or in and behind the eye.

Picture a long dining room table with a white table cloth. Perhaps the table is set for Thanksgiving dinner. Imagine pulling slowly but firmly on one corner only. Can you picture a wrinkle formed the entire length of the table cloth? Even though all dishes move, they do so less and less the farther away you move from the area that you pull.

Now, picture your head balanced on the spinal column. Can you see how a hip out of place could, just like the table cloth, "wrinkle" the muscles all the way up the back and neck into the head and ultimately, the TMJs? Now you can begin to understand how bad posture, injury to the neck or even the hips can influence the head and TMJs.

We often see patients with their head thrust forward and their chin tilted up. This usually occurs with those who have a small lower jaw or who have had a neck injury. This posture also happens in those who sit for hours at a computer or typewriter.

Forward head posture causes the mandible to close differently than it should, thus causing malocclusion (*bad bite*). This in turn may trigger the person to grind or clench his or her teeth. This forward head posture also causes tension in the muscles of the neck and back, producing head, neck and back pain. Frequently, these painful muscles refer pain into the head, face and TMJs, causing both patient and doctor to think that the pain is coming from the TMJs. Can you see how confusing the process of diagnosing pain can be?

The diagnosis and treatment of pain can be quite complex and misdiagnoses may be common.

The names of the neck and back muscles aren't really important. However, the effect from increased tension in these muscles is important. If our balance is disturbed for any length of time, we can experience head, facial and TMJ pain without these structures really being physically injured. So you can see that the diagnosis and treatment of pain can be quite complex and misdiagnoses may be common.

Two

Symptoms of TMJ

Because there are so many different symptoms of TMJ, making a proper diagnosis is difficult. However, there are a few classic symptoms that involve the TM joints, ears, head, face and teeth.

Temporomandibular Joints

The most common symptom of TMJ is jaw joint clicking (popping, snapping) or locking. This clicking sound may be so loud that it can be heard by others while you chew. The noise is actually produced by the cartilage disc being caught between the two bones of the TMJ as the lower jaw moves.

There may or may not be pain in the joint itself with the sound of a click or pop. But one thing is for sure: If there is a displaced disc, as is usually the case when a click occurs, then the muscles that move the jaw while chewing are more tense than normal. This tenseness can and does cause muscle, facial, head and neck pain.

Locking of the TMJs may feel like a catching of the lower jaw as it opens. Sometimes, the person with a locked joint must move the jaw to one side or another in order to open wide. Or a person might have to open until he hears and feels a loud pop, at which point the jaw actually unlocks. As with clicking, there may or may not be pain associated with locking. If the locking is a result of injury to the head or jaw, pain almost always occurs.

A dislocated TMJ may also be noticed by a change in the dental *occlusion*, or bite. If the TMJ disc goes out of place, the bones and disc do not fit together properly and therefore, the bite of the teeth changes.

One last comment about a dislocated TMJ disc: the TMJ can actually lock wide open. This is a very terrifying experience. It usually occurs after a wide opening movement such as a yawn. However, an open lock of the TMJ can also occur after a long dental appointment, being put to sleep for any type of surgery, or even after opening wide to eat an apple or large sandwich. Open locking that occurs again and again is a sign of weak or loose TMJ ligaments. We often see this in teenage girls limber enough to perform as cheerleaders or gymnasts.

If a patient has seen many different doctors and therapists, has taken all types of medication, has tried all sorts of exercises and still the headache pain persists, then a TMJ problem should be highly suspected.

Ears

Due to the close relationship of the TMJs and ears, an injury to the TMJ often causes ear symptoms. Some of the symptoms are pain, fullness or stuffiness, and even a loss of hearing. That is why many TMJ sufferers first go to their family doctor and then to an ear doctor for help. Usually, an examination of the ear is normal, even if there appears to be a loss of hearing. Patients may take several different types of antibiotics because of the fullness in the ears, even in the absence of other symptoms that usually signal an infection (fever, redness, heat, discharge).

Head

Headache is one of the most common symptoms of a TMJ problem. Although any area of the head may be affected, usually the TMJ headache is located in the temples, back of the head, and even the shoulders.

Clenching and grinding of the teeth, both of which themselves may be TMJ symptoms, produce muscle pain which can cause headache pain. Also, a displaced disc in the TMJ may cause pain in the joint that is often referred into the temples, forehead or neck. These headaches are frequently so severe that they are confused and treated (with little success) as migraine headaches or abnormalities in the brain.

Normal healthy muscles are not generally tender. Tender areas in these muscles [of the face, neck or shoulders] may indicate TMJ.

If a patient has seen many doctors and therapists, has taken all types of medication, has tried all sorts of exercises and still the headache pain persists, then a TMJ problem should be highly suspected. These unfortunate patients often have had numerous x-rays, CAT scans and MRIs. No diagnosis is found, and worse yet, they continue to suffer.

Face

Anatomically, our faces have more nerves than nearly all other areas of our bodies. Psychologically, we as humans are known by our faces. Although we often attempt to hide our true feelings by wearing a disguise, it is virtually impossible to hide the private experience of pain. When we hurt, our faces show pain. Also, pain from the TMJ may be referred to the face even though the TMJ itself does not really hurt. Facial pain may be deep in the face or on the surface of the skin. The skin might even become sensitive to the touch or air blowing over it. Often, a neurologist is seen for this type of pain.

Teeth

A displaced TMJ disc may cause tooth pain. The teeth may become sensitive to temperatures, especially cold. The teeth may also become sensitive because of jaw activities such as clenching of the teeth or grinding of the teeth. Patients may see their dentist for pain in the teeth, but the dentist can find no cause. Frequently (and very unfortunately), unnecessary root canals and even tooth extractions are performed in an attempt to help a suffering person. What's worse, after these invasive and non-reversible procedures, patients still have their pain, only now it has increased!

Other symptoms

Many other symptoms may be associated with TMJ. Often, pain will be felt in the shoulders and back due to muscle contraction (a condition called myofascial pain dysfunction syndrome, which will be discussed later). Dizziness, disorientation and even confusion are also seen in some people who suffer with TMJ.

Depression is common with TMJ. This may be because no one really believes this problem causes such pain and suffering. Also, plenty of scientific evidence shows that chronic pain patients (which includes most TMJ patients) have changes in chemicals in the brain (termed neurotransmitters) as a result of the pain. These chemicals can and do produce depression.

Along with depression comes an inability to get a good night's sleep. This may be due to TMJ pain itself or changes in the brain's neurotransmitters, which produce stimulation even though the TMJ sufferer is asleep. Sufferers often wake feeling like they never slept. This lack of sleep not only makes their pain seem worse, but also adds fuel to the fire of depression.

A TMJ patient may also suffer with *photophobia,* or light sensitivity. A dislocated TMJ may produce pain in and behind the eye which can cause sensitivity to light. Blurred vision and eye muscle twitching are also common in TMJ patients.

Another common symptom, and one that prompted Dr. Costen in the 1930s to first write about TMJ, is ringing (termed *tinnitus*) in the ears. This sound may be caused by many different problems (such as working around loud noises or taking too much aspirin or ibuprofen). Yet, it is one symptom that I personally see in about 60% of all TMJ patients.

Questions to Ask Yourself

At this point, it might be helpful to examine a few questions that you can ask yourself, just to see if you may be one of those suffering from TMJ or a related disorder. Remember, an accurate diagnosis can't be made based on answers to questions alone. However, positive answers may help indicate if you or someone you know should seek professional advice.

Table 1. Questions about your symptoms

1. Do you have frequent headaches?
2. Do you hear popping, clicking or cracking sounds when you chew?
3. Do you hear a grating sound (like crumpling of newspaper) when you chew?
4. Do you have stuffiness, pressure or blockage in your ears?
5. Do you hear a ringing or buzzing sound in either or both of your ears?
6. Do you experience dizziness frequently?
7. Do your jaws feel like they "catch?"
8. Do your jaws feel tight, difficult to open?
9. Does it appear that you can't open your mouth as wide as you used to?
10. Does your tongue go between your teeth or do you bite on your tongue to separate your teeth?

Table 1. Questions about your symptoms *(cont)*

11. Do your teeth ache?
12. Are your teeth sensitive, especially to cold temperatures?
13. Do you wake with sore facial muscles?
14. Do you clench or grind your teeth during moments of frustration or concentration?
15. Do you grind your teeth at night?
16. Do your ears hurt?
17. Does it hurt to move your jaw sideways?
18. Do your neck, back of your head, or shoulder hurt?
19. Have you been hit in the jaw?
20. Have you been put to sleep for surgery?
21. Have you had a whiplash injury?
22. Have you seen a neurologist, chiropractor, psychologist or psychiatrist for unexplained head or neck pain?
23. Do your jaws ache after eating?
24. Are you under a lot of stress?
25. Have you been told that you might have TMJ?

If you answered "Yes" to any of the questions on the list, you might be suffering with some form of TMJ. Before you make a doctor's appointment, perform the self-examination listed next. Remember, the more "Yes" answers that you have increases the odds that you might be suffering with TMJ.

Self-examination for TMJ

A TMJ self-exam is easy to perform in just a few moments. As always, remember that positive findings with the self-examination do not necessarily mean that you are suffering from TMJ. If you have several "Yes" answers and several positive exam results, it might be well worth your time to see a TMJ specialist. *How to find a TMJ specialist is listed in a Chapter 14.*

Jaw movements

- Looking directly into a wall mirror, slowly open and close your mouth. Watch to see if your jaw moves in a straight line or if it seems to move to one side or another. Watch this movement both with opening and closing. With a normal, uninjured TMJ, the lower jaw should move in a straight line both when opening and when closing.

- With your mouth open, you should be able to get approximately three fingers between your front upper and lower teeth (Figure 6).

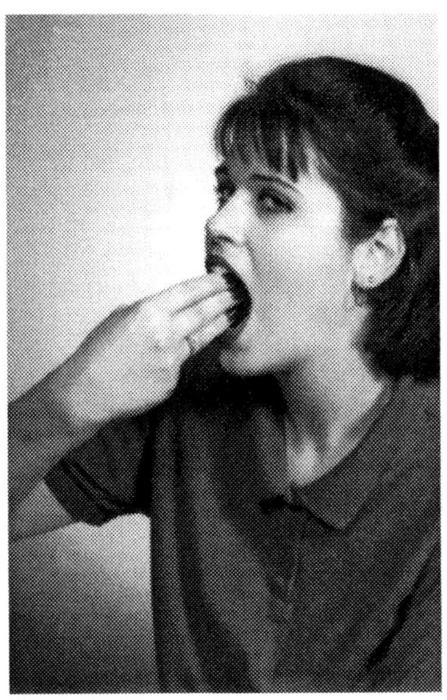

Figure 6. Normal mouth opening

- Also, with your mouth open just a little, move your jaw both to the left and then to the right. These movements should be about the same. With practice, there should be little confusion as to which side you are attempting to move.
- Lastly, move your lower jaw forward. You should be able to bring the lower jaw forward in a straight line. If any of these movements do not appear to be normal, then you might have a TMJ problem.

Listen for TMJ noises

In a quiet room, open and close your mouth several times. Do you hear any type of noise? You should be listening for a popping or clicking sound. You might even hear a crunching or *crepitation* sound. If you can hear a noise, once again look in the mirror. Notice if the lower jaw moves or deviates to one side when opening as the noise is heard. If you can hear any of these noises, you might have a TMJ problem.

Pain. Do you experience pain with wide opening of your mouth, with side to side or forward movements of your jaw? Place your fingers over your TMJs, just in front of your ears, and gently push and notice if either or both joints are sore or tender (Figure 7). If you place your little fingers in your ear canals and gently push forward do your TMJs hurt? (Figure 8)

Do the TMJs hurt when you close hard on your back teeth and squeeze? If so, does placing a tissue between your back teeth and then squeezing stop the pain? Any of these activities that produce pain should alert you to the possibility of a TMJ problem. Remember: normal joints do not hurt. Push on your shoulder or knee. Do they hurt? They won't if they are healthy.

Push on your face. Look in the mirror and push firmly on all the muscles in your face and along your lower jaw. Healthy muscles do not hurt. If you notice

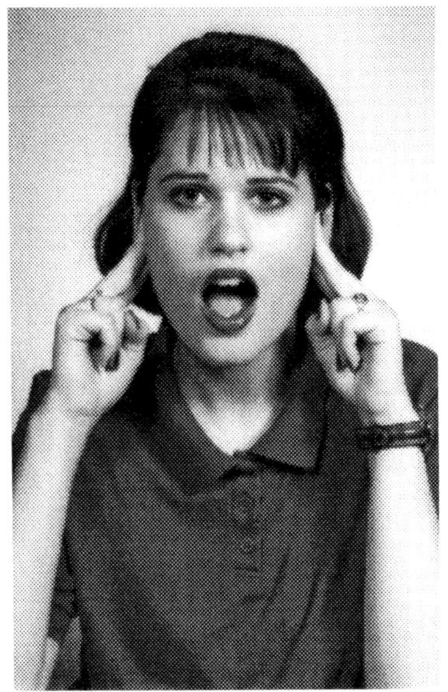

Figure 7: Palpating the TMJ

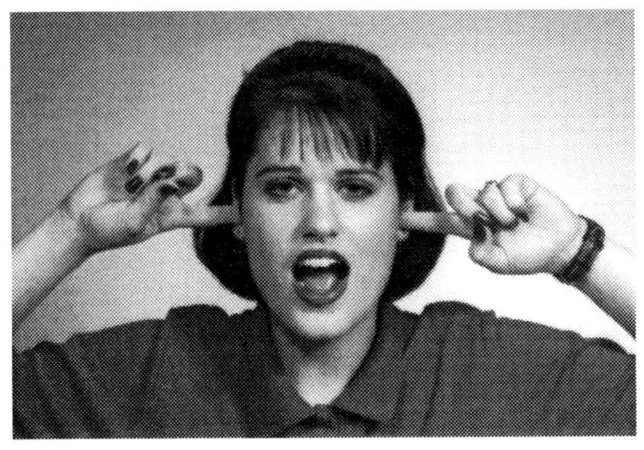

Figure 8: Palpation of the TMJs through the ear canal

a tender area, this may indicate soreness caused by TMJ.

Feel your neck and upper back muscles. Firmly push against your neck muscles at the attachment of your neck with your head. Are there tender spots? If you sit at a computer, typewriter, or work as a painter or hair stylist, then you might be experiencing an occupational hazard and not a TMJ problem. Feel your neck lower down; feel your shoulders. Are there tender areas? Again, normal healthy muscles are not generally tender. Tender areas in these muscles may indicate TMJ.

Abnormal jaw movements or TMJ noises may indicate a TMJ problem.

A few positive findings (noises or some tender areas) may be normal, especially if you are middle aged or older. However, an inability to open wide enough for at least 2½ fingers to be placed between your front teeth, a gross deviation to one side while opening your mouth, pain with joint noises and numerous tender areas in the facial and neck muscles are all specific symptoms of TMJ. Couple these symptoms with suffering from undiagnosed head, neck or facial pain, and positive answers to several questions, and you might see a developing profile of a TMJ sufferer.

Pain and Activity Diary

If you keep a daily diary, then you might be able to determine if there is a pattern to your symptoms. Are there any environmental factors (for example, physical activities, stress, chewing, certain foods or drinks, etc.) that cause your pain and other symptoms? Do you remember what symptoms you have or how long they last? How severe are your symptoms and are there any associated triggers?

Copy the diary on the last two pages of this chapter and make at least seven copies so that you can chart your symptoms for one week. Try to see any patterns (for example, foods or drinks that may appear to produce pain symptoms). Diaries are very important in determining if there are environmental factors contributing to your pain symptoms. Keep an accurate record of your symptoms and record any information immediately. In other words, keep the diary up to date.

Healthy muscles and TMJs don't hurt.

Chances are good that you'll see a pattern. If you do, then try to make appropriate changes to see if your symptoms improve. When consulting any type of doctor, provide him or her with a copy of your diary — it should be of great help in determining your diagnosis and recommended treatment.

Time of Day	Symptoms	Severity*	Activities	Food/ Drink	Meds**
Morning 6:00 - 6:30					
6:30 - 7:00					
7:00 - 7:30					
7:30 - 8:00					
8:00 - 8:30					
8:30 - 9:00					
9:00 - 9:30					
9:30 - 10:00					
10:00- 10:30					
10:30 - 11:00					
11:00 - 11:30					
11:30 - noon					
Afternoon noon - 12:30					
12:30 - 1:00					
1:00 - 1:30					
1:30 - 2:00					
2:00 - 2:30					
2:30 - 3:00					

*Severity of symptoms graded 0 to 10: 0 = no pain; 5 = moderate pain; 10 = unbearable pain.

Time of Day	Symptoms	Severity*	Activities	Food/ Drink	Meds**
Afternoon 3:00 - 3:30					
3:30 - 4:00					
4:00 - 4:30					
4:30 - 5:00					
5:00 - 5:30					
5:30 - 6:00					
Evening 6:00 - 6:30					
6:30 - 7:00					
7:00 - 7:30					
7:30 - 8:00					
8:00 - 8:30					
8:30 - 9:00					
9:00 - 9:30					
9:30 - 10:00					
10:00 - 10:30					
10:30 - 11:00					
11:00 - 11:30					
11:30 - midnight					

**Meds: Any prescription or non-prescription (over-the-counter) medications.

Three

What Causes TMJ?

"Your eyes only see what your brain knows."

That saying is certainly true when it comes to the cause or causes of TMJ. For years dentists believed that malocclusion (a bad bite) was the chief cause of TMJ. Chiropractic physicians and physical therapists have been taught that muscle problems and poor posture are the cause for TMJ. Nutritionists contend that poor nutrition may be a major contributing factor, and medical doctors list stress as the main cause.

Guess what? They're all correct!

Many problems can contribute to problems within any joint, but one thing is for sure: there are many different causes. At times, only one major cause can be found. On other occasions, many factors may contribute to the development of a TMJ problem.

Internal Joint Derangements

What in the world are internal joint derangements? When we speak of specific TMJ damage or injury, we mean a problem within the joint itself. A derangement in orthopedic terms simply means a disturbance in the regular order or arrangement. Therefore, internal derangements of the TMJ are disturbances in the arrangement of the components within the joint itself, primarily the disc. Internal derangements are the most common disorders of the TMJ.

There are many different types of internal derangements of the TMJ. The most common is a clicking joint; another is a locking joint. Derangements occur in all joints. The difference with the TMJ is that the articular disc actually moves with normal jaw movement, acting like a third bone.

Normally, the disc is located between the mandibular condyle and the temporal bone of the skull (Figure 9) with the disc between the bones, on top of the condyle. In the most common internal derangement, an anterior dislocation of the disc, the disc slips forward with a subsequent posterior displacement of the condyle. As the mouth is opened, a "click" occurs when the disc is caught between the bones (Fig. 9). This catching of the disc between the bones is not always heard, but it can be felt. A click in the TMJ might also be felt and heard as the opened mouth closes. This opening and closing click is termed reciprocal clicking.

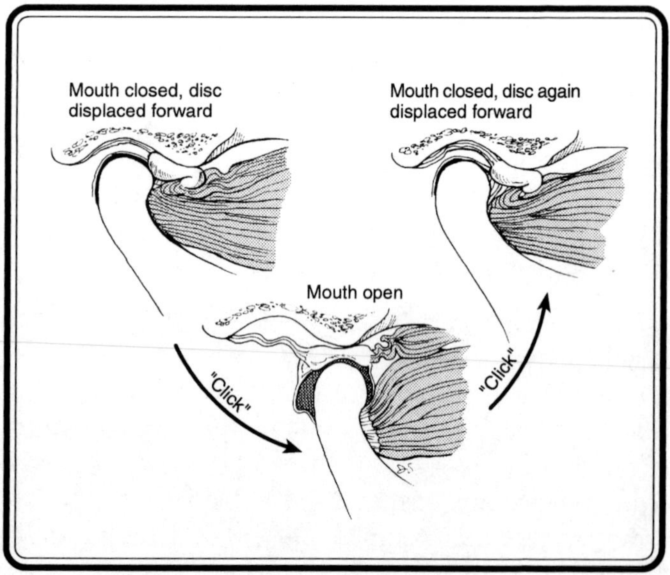

Figure 9: Displaced TMJ disc

As time goes on, the clicking will either subside or get worse. If worse, there is a good chance that the jaw will ultimately lock, usually closed. Closed locking of the TMJ can be extremely painful and certainly can be terrifying.

The symptoms of early locking of the TMJ can usually be treated rather successfully. However, once clicking and then locking occur, these internal derangements are permanent. Even if your pain can be reduced or eliminated, the internal derangement still exists and will remain for the rest of your life.

Some of the conditions blamed for internal derangements of the TMJ are: trauma, opening the mouth too wide, bruxism, malocclusion, ligament laxity, stress, and arthritis.

Another internal derangement of the TMJ is arthritis. Like all other synovial joints (those that produce synovial fluid for lubrication), the TMJ can undergo changes on the surface of its bones producing an arthritic condition. This problem is treated just like arthritis of other joints: moist heat, rest, physical therapy and medication.

What are the common causes of internal derangements of the TMJ? There are many. Some of the conditions blamed are: trauma, opening the mouth too wide, bruxism, malocclusion, orthodontics, ligament laxity and stress. In addition, certain systemic diseases may produce a TMJ problem.

Trauma

According to statistics published in the Journal of the American Dental Association in 1991, 44% to 99% of TMJ problems are caused by trauma. By trauma, we mean an injury as obvious as a blow to the jaw with a fist or something as subtle as a whiplash injury with or without direct trauma to the head or jaw. As you will recall, the lower jaw is connected to the upper jaw by a series of ligaments and muscles.

Remember that the disc in the TMJ is held in its proper place by tiny, fragile ligaments. A direct blow to the jaw with a fist, baseball bat, or hitting the steering wheel in an accident may drive the lower jaw upwards and back, thus stretching or tearing these tiny ligaments (Figure 10). A frequent result is a dislocated disc producing TMJ.

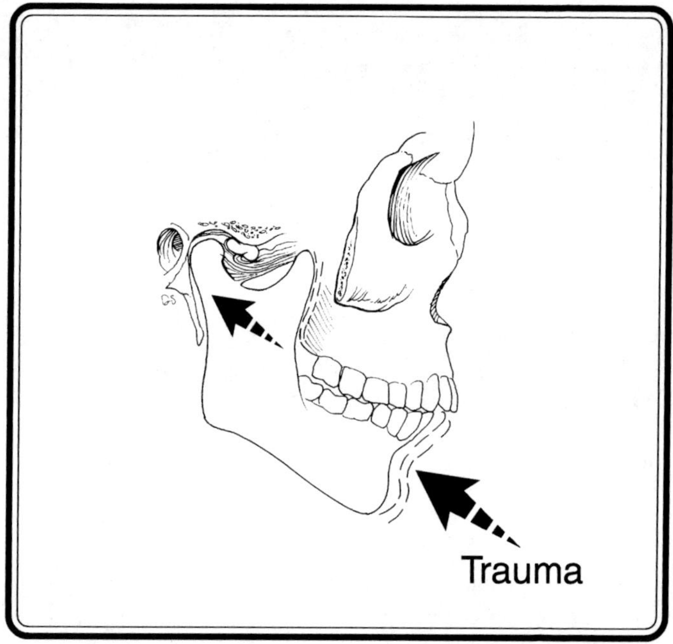

Figure 10: Trauma causing TMJ injury

This same process occurs in other joints. You certainly know someone who has twisted his or her knee or ankle, tearing ligaments and injuring the joint. If ligaments aren't torn after trauma, the joints can at least be bruised. In the TMJ, this bruising produces swelling, a change in the bite, and even ear and headache pain. If the swelling is severe and left untreated, the disc may gradually be displaced and a click may develop.

Opening Too Wide

All joints have limitations to movement and the TMJ is no exception. If you open wide for a long time, or if your mouth is forced wide open, ligaments may be torn. Swelling and bruising develop and disc dislocation may occur. For example, if your mouth is open for a long time at the dental office while having a tooth prepared for a crown, the joint can dislocate. This rarely happens without a prior history of clicking; however, it does happen. Also, this type of injury may occur if someone's mouth is opened too wide when they are being put to sleep for surgery. Again, both of these examples are accidental and consequences of the given procedures.

Most of us grind our teeth and clench our jaws at times, but if it continues, TMJ injury might occur.

Bruxism

What in the world is bruxism? Bruxism is abnormal grinding of the teeth. Anyone who has had a small child knows that horrible sound of teeth grinding at nighttime — worse than fingernails on a blackboard!

If grinding continues or develops later in life, TMJ may develop. Bruxism usually occurs during sleep. That is why so many people do not realize that they are bruxers. Most of us brux at one time or another. But if this activity continues for any length of time, then symptoms develop.

One indication that a person is a bruxer is sore jaw muscles when waking in the morning. Some researchers feel that the constant grinding of the teeth causing pressure on the TMJs may injure the ligaments, thus allowing the disc to dislocate. At the very least, bruxism produces muscle pain sensitivity, and worn teeth.

Clenching is a form of bruxism that can also cause TMJ. Clenching may occur at any time. However, it is most noticeable during times of frustration, concentration or stress. Again, some think that the constant pressures applied to the joints from chronic clenching stretch or injure the ligaments, thereby producing a TMJ problem.

Double-jointed people (especially women) tend to be predisposed to TMJ problems.

Malocclusion

One additional cause of TMJ is malocclusion, or a bad bite. Malocclusion may be produced by poor development of the jaws or removal of teeth without replacement. Malocclusion may also be caused by a high dental restoration, a poor fitting denture or partial denture, or a displaced TMJ disc.

Malocclusion may be one cause of bruxism: The bite being off, the brain tends to make a person grind his or her teeth to even the bite, thus reducing the malocclusion. This becomes a vicious cycle: Malocclusion produces bruxism; bruxism produces sore muscles and sensitive teeth; and sore muscles and sensitive teeth can produce malocclusion.

One important comment must be made about malocclusion. Virtually every dentist believes that malocclusion can cause a TMJ problem. However, there has never been a scientifically controlled study to prove this concept.

Orthodontics

Some dentists feel that orthodontic treatment, or braces, might be a cause of TMJ. By moving teeth with orthodontic appliances, malocclusion is produced during treatment. Also, people undergoing orthodontics do report sensitive teeth, pain in the jaw muscles and even bruxism. However, as with malocclusion, there has been no adequate controlled studies that prove that orthodontic treatment produces a TMJ problem. In fact, there have been several recent studies demonstrating that orthodontic treatment may prevent TMJ problems from starting. The jury is still out on this controversial issue. I myself have seen no correlation with orthodontically treated patients and those suffering with TMJ.

Ligament Laxity

Stress exacerbates TMJ problems like gasoline thrown on an existing fire.

We all remember fellow classmates that appeared to be double-jointed, meaning that they could bend their fingers back really far or they could put one leg behind their head and so on. Many of these kids became cheerleaders or gymnasts because they were so limber. They were not double-jointed; they actually suffered from a problem termed ligament laxity. If you will also recall, most were girls. This is because women have a hormone that is released from their pituitary gland (relaxin), which helps in the birth of children. If a young or teenaged girl happens to have a little more of this hormone than normal, and if she also put a lot of stress on joints (in such activities as cheer-leading and gymnastics), then her ligaments do not preserve the tightness of a joint. If this occurs, then the joint appears to be double or loose.

This definitely can happen to the TMJs. Ligament laxity is a fairly common problem in active young women who suffer with TMJ (and injuries to other joints).

A disease called Ehlers-Danlos syndrome is a connective tissue disorder that is characterized by joint hypermobility. Sometimes the skin becomes extensible (stretchable) and tissue becomes fragile. These patients frequently experience chronic musculoskeletal pain affecting many joints, including the TMJ.

Stress

Does stress have an effect on the TMJ? Not unless you're alive!

Stress has many effects on our bodies, some good and some bad. Stress, being both physical and psychological, produces an increase in certain chemicals in the blood (catecholamines). These chemicals cause tenseness, restlessness, stimulation and an increase in blood pressure. Blood vessels on the surface of the body constrict and skeletal muscles become tight and develop painful regions termed trigger points.

All of these physiological changes can produce muscle tightness and pain. These physical changes are good if you need a "fight or flight" response when faced with a stressful situation. However, if you are subjected to chronic stress, these physical changes may produce harmful effects. For example, people subjected to chronic stress develop ulcers, diarrhea, tension headaches, muscle tightness and other physical symptoms.

Now, add these changes to an existing TMJ problem, even one that is hardly noticeable, and a very painful situation can occur. It is just like throwing gasoline on an existing fire, where the fire is a TMJ problem and the gasoline is stress. The gasoline causes the fire to flair up and burn widely for a time, but the gasoline did not produce the fire (or TMJ), it just made it worse.

This is how stress can exacerbate a TMJ problem. Muscles tighten, teeth clench, abnormal pressure is forced against the TMJ disc, and if the ligaments are weak or if the patient has ligament laxity, then the disc may dislocate.

Systemic Diseases

Various diseases can cause or aggravate TMJ problems. Immune disorders such as rheumatoid arthritis, psoriatic arthritis, and systemic lupus erythematosus can produce inflammation in the TMJ. In addition, viral infections such as mononucleosis, mumps and measles can cause damage to the surfaces of the TMJ, which ultimately can lead to an internal derangement.

Miscellaneous

Normal, everyday activities can sometimes cause TMJ pain. Musicians who play woodwind, brass, and string instruments may need to wear a bite splint and to limit the length of playing time in order to relieve pain in the jaw. Violin players experience less pain when they use a rack as shoulder support for their instrument.

A report in the New England Journal of Medicine described a woman with "headphone neuralgia," who developed TMJ symptoms while using hard plastic headphone earpieces in the auditory canal. Her symptoms subsided when she switched to "earmuff" type earpieces.

People whose work involves abnormal head and neck positions may develop TMJ pain. So, for example, if you routinely perform car repairs, you may be at risk.

Vocal musicians may have TMJ symptoms that will affect their singing voice. Singers have reported that their endurance, tone quality/resonance, vibrato, legato and staccato are often affected, along with posture difficulties and problems with diction.

The self-help measures in Chapter 11 may be sufficient to return a singer to his or her former capacity. For example, you may need to consciously remind yourself to unclench your jaw if you find your self clenching, and breathe through your nose when not singing or talking. Avoid opening your jaw too wide. Use a soft diet when necessary, and avoid caffeine and sugar.

Four

Diagnosis of TMJ

The best service any doctor can give his or her patient is an accurate diagnosis. Often, and especially with TMJ, patients travel from office to office in an attempt to find an answer for their pain problems.

In 1983, we studied the medical histories of 135 patients who were referred to our office for TMJ. Of all those patients, our office was the 6th, on average, visited in search of relief of pain.

Would you take your car to a garage just hoping that the mechanic had the proper training? Then why go to a doctor who may know nothing about TMJ?

Can you imagine traveling to five or six different service stations or having five or six different plumbers to your house for a stopped-up drain? In each of these cases, the mechanic or plumber would charge a fee for his time (which he should) but he would never tell you what was wrong. Does that make sense? Of course not! To make matters worse, the mechanic would replace several different parts on your car, but he really wouldn't know if any of them would help your engine problems. How long would you stand for such "service?" And yet, on average, I was the sixth doctor whom these unfortunate people consulted for pain. Obviously, something was wrong.

I cannot claim that all of these patients' complaints were identified or successfully treated under my care. However, very specific diagnostic procedures were followed and a diagnosis was found. Every TMJ sufferer deserves the same.

An accurate diagnosis demands that you be examined by a physician trained in the diagnosis and treatment of TMJ. This doctor, usually a dentist, may also be a medical doctor, a chiropractor, or an osteopathic physician.

Not all doctors even believe that TMJ exists, let alone know how to diagnose problems with these complex joints. Therefore, it's important that you ask the receptionist when you make an appointment for an examination if the doctor (1) treats TMJ problems, and (2) what type of credentials he or she might have.

When you make an appointment for an examination if the doctor (1) treats TMJ problems, and (2) what type of credentials he or she might have.

Would you take your car to a garage just hoping that the mechanic had the proper training? Then why go to a doctor who may know nothing about TMJ?

Medical History

When you arrive for your first appointment, does the doctor have a detailed medical history form to be completed? Will this doctor review the answers on the medical history form, listen to you, and take you seriously? If the doctor does not take time to talk with you, or if he or she seems to make light of TMJ problems, then you are probably wasting time and money.

What actually is a detailed medical history? A detailed history is composed of many different questions. These questions should ask specifically about your complaints (symptoms). For example, how long have you had pain? Where is the pain? Does it radiate to other sites? What type of pain do you have (dull, sharp, deep, aching, etc.)? Do your TMJs click or pop? Do your TMJs ever lock? Do you have headaches?

The doctor (or at times an assistant or nurse) should ask you to demonstrate exactly where the pain originates and then where it radiates. You should be asked just how long the pain lasts and if the intensity varies. The doctor will be interested in any activity that makes the pain worse or better. You might also be asked to rate the pain on a scale (0 = no pain; 10 = the most intense pain you can stand) as to the average severity.

Physical Examination

After your medical history is reviewed, a physical examination should then be performed. The exam will probably take several minutes and will consist of several different sections.

Vital signs. Usually the assistant or nurse will take your blood pressure, pulse and temperature. Many people suffer with headaches and a clicking TMJ only to actually have high blood pressure and not a TMJ problems that needs to be treated. By taking your blood pressure, the office staff can begin the process of diagnosis. In other words, do you really suffer with TMJ alone or do you have a secondary (and perhaps more serious) problem?

Posture. Your posture should also be evaluated. Believe it or not, "The leg bone is connected to the back bone." Poor posture may have a dramatic effect on the TMJs. It may be a result of a back injury or a result of a bad TMJ problem. In our office, the staff observes the gait (walking) of all patients without their knowledge. This gives us a lot of information concerning posture. We also notice the patient's head position in respect to the rest of the body.

TMJ examination. Your TMJs should be evaluated by the doctor. Palpation (feeling and pushing) over and around the joints is performed to determine if the joints are sore or painful.

Also, you will be asked to open your mouth and the opening will be measured. The average opening of healthy TMJs should be around 40 millimeters to 55 millimeters (1½ to 2¼ inches). If the joints are healthy, there should be normal opening without pain, noise, or deviation to one side or the other.

Next, lateral movement of the lower jaw will be measured. The average lateral movement of healthy TMJs is approximately 9 millimeters to 14 or 15 millimeters. Again, there should be no pain, noise or catching if the joints are healthy.

By taking the extra effort to listen to the sounds of the joint, invaluable information may be learned to help in establishing an accurate diagnosis and later, proper treatment.

Forward movement of the lower jaw will be measured. The average forward movement should be about 5 to 7 or 8 millimeters, with no pain or catching.

The doctor next will probably closely examine the movement of your TMJs. He or she will place his or her fingers over the joints and ask you to open and close. The doctor can feel the movement of the joints as your mouth opens. This maneuver will produce a lot of information. Snapping or clicking can usually be felt; deviation of the jaw with opening can also be detected. Also, by palpating the joints with opening movements, a joint that may seem healthy might feel tender with the doctor's pressure being applied.

No TMJ examination is complete without listening to the joints either with a stethoscope, an ultrasound device, or both. These instruments can demonstrate sounds in the joints that might not be audible to the doctor or even the patient. Joint noises are very diagnostic for specific internal problems. By taking the extra effort to listen to the sounds of the joint, invaluable information may be learned to help in establishing an accurate diagnosis and later, proper treatment.

A deeper look at the TMJs. Depending upon the severity of your problem, the doctor will probably order certain types of x-rays of the joints. A common x-ray, taken around your head, is known as a panoramic x-ray. This x-ray is not very good for evaluating the TMJs except in cases of severe arthritis, fractures or tumors.

Those who treat TMJ problems usually order a transcranial x-ray. This specialized view shows the bony surfaces of the TMJs. It also gives some information concerning the position of the lower jaw in the joint.

The doctor might also order a very special (and expensive) image called a Magnetic Resonance Image or MRI. This technique, unlike x-rays, shows the soft tissue of the joints (muscles, ligaments, disc, etc.). Although an MRI is a very accurate way to view the position of the disc within the TMJ, this test is not usually necessary unless the doctor is considering surgery as a choice of treatment.

Although an MRI is a very accurate way to view the position of the disc within the TMJ, this test is not usually necessary unless the doctor is considering surgery as a choice of treatment.

The most accurate x-ray view of the temporomandibular joints is obtained by taking corrected tomograms. This specific x-ray technique is difficult but well worth the effort. Seeing the precise position of the lower jaw with this view gives the doctor a good idea about the position of the articular disc. Also, the bony surfaces of the joint can be studied.

Impressions. After obtaining the above information, the doctor will often order impressions (or molds) of your teeth and jaws in order to study how they bite together. Abnormal wear and improper contacts of the teeth are also demonstrated by studying the models made from the impressions.

Blood tests. At times, certain blood tests might be recommended. The values determined from blood tests might indicate a disease that may or may not cause a problem in the TMJs.

Consultation with other doctors. Your doctor may want to consult with other health care professionals. Often, patients feel abandoned when referred to another doctor. Actually, this is a sign of humility and honesty on the part of the doctor. Any doctor who feels that he or she can do everything without help from others should be avoided. If your doctor wishes to refer you for a consultation to someone else, this usually means that another point of view is necessary. This is quite different from you, on your own, traveling from office to office without direction. Instead of your wandering in search for help, by referring you, the doctor is guiding your exploration.

Patients may feel abandoned when referred to another doctor. Actually, this is a sign of humility and honesty on the part of the doctor.

Five

Treatment of TMJ

The treatment of TMJ has always been controversial. Since dentists are the experts of the jaws, teeth, TMJs and other structures in the head, it is natural that they would provide the most care for TMJ. However, chiropractors, medical doctors, physical and masso-therapists also contribute to treatment of these disorders. But usually, dentists treat TMJ.

What Is Successful Treatment?

What would you, as a sufferer of TMJ or a related disorder, consider successful treatment? Some would demand total relief of pain. Others might feel that 50% reduction of pain is reasonable. The answer depends upon the type and amount of suffering that one is experiencing. The patient must make this decision in concert with his or her family and with the doctor. Is it realistic to expect total relief or is this only a hope?

As a doctor who treats those who endure these disorders, I can only say that most soft tissue injuries, such as all those under the term of TMJ, have the potential for re-injury and recurrence of pain. This statement is realistic and yet frightening to some. It need not be.

If one understands that there are limitations in activities once a TMJ problem has occurred, then one can reasonably live with less pain, and sometimes none. However, I can't state strongly enough that it is totally unrealistic to assume that pain and dysfunction will never recur. Broken bones and teeth can heal or be mended; soft tissues do not enjoy such luxury.

Treatment Modalities

Dentists use a variety of treatment modalities, which may be divided into Phase I and Phase II therapy. The purpose of Phase I therapy is to eliminate muscle spasms, TMJ swelling and dislocation (if possible), and generally reduce any type of pain. This treatment usually includes the use of splints, exercises, medication, injections of local anesthetics or other medications, physical therapy and chiropractic treatment.

The purpose of Phase I therapy is to eliminate muscle spasms, TMJ swelling and dislocation (if possible), and generally reduce any type of pain.

The purpose of Phase II therapy is to definitively correct any discrepancies, if necessary, between the upper and lower jaws. Phase II therapy may include adjustment of the dental occlusion, orthodontics, reconstruction of the teeth, surgery, or a combination of some of the above treatments. It is important to note that Phase II therapy should not be attempted without successful Phase I therapy modalities.

Phase I Therapy

Phase I therapy is usually composed of two types of treatment, both aimed at reducing or eliminating muscle and joint pain:

1. The use of an intraoral splint
2. The use of different modes of treatment to reduce muscle pain.

Phase I therapy is considered reversible. In other words, if treatment is discontinued, no detrimental changes will have occurred. If patients see no

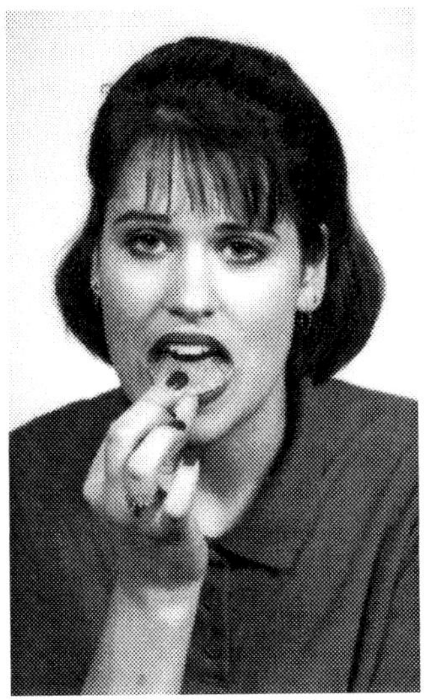

Figure 11. Upper splint

improvement, then they are no worse off than before they began treatment.

Splints. The use of a splint is the primary treatment for most TMJ disorders. A splint (also known as an appliance, a bite plane or an orthotic) is usually a clear plastic mouthpiece similar to an orthodontic retainer. It is usually worn in the mouth for 24 hours a day for several months or even years. Splints may be placed on either the upper or lower teeth.

There are three categories of splints. The first type is a *superior repositioning appliance.* The primarily purpose of this splint is to relax the muscles and take pressure off the TMJs so that inflammation subsides. This type is worn at all times for periods up to six or eight months. If the patient does well and feels significantly better, he or she is usually weaned off the splint so that ultimately, it is worn just at night or during times of intense concentration or stress.

A second category of splint might be termed an *anterior repositioning appliance.* This splint brings the lower jaw forward and is used when one or both TMJs are dislocating (clicking and/or locking). It too removes pressure from the joints so that inflammation can subside. This splint must be worn even when chewing.

A third type of splint is an *anti-bruxism splint.* It is worn primarily when sleeping in order to reduce bruxism or its effects. At times, this type of splint might also be worn during the day when a person is subjected to stress. Everyone bruxes from time to time. However, the medical literature states that approximately 35% of all people will continue to brux no matter what treatment is given. This appliance simply counteracts the bad effects of bruxism such as muscle pain, tooth wear, tooth sensitivity and even injury to the TMJs.

Often, I see patients who have had splints before. Many times an improper type of splint has previously been used. So don't be surprised if your TMJ doctor recommends a splint even though you've had one before.

Often, I see patients who have had splints before. They may not understand why I would order yet another. The answer is rather simple. Many times an improper type of splint was used before. If we can, a patient's existing splint will be used. However, don't be surprised if your TMJ doctor recommends a splint even though you've already had one (or two or three or...) before.

Medication. Often, medications are used to simply cover up symptoms. Yet, there are times when medication, used properly and conservatively, is very beneficial.

Various medications are used for different reasons. For example, aspirin is still the medication of choice for pain and inflammation. Also, ibuprofen (Motrin) is a good drug for treating these two problems.

Acetaminophen (Tylenol) is equally good for pain management but unfortunately, this chemical does not have an effect on inflammation. However, this pain medication is kinder to the stomach than aspirin or ibuprofen and is often prescribed for patients that have ulcers or stomach problems. Also, aspirin and ibuprofen, taken for a long time, can produce ringing in the ears and bleeding problems. Long-term use of acetaminophen is not without problems — this drug can produce kidney damage. None of these medications should be taken for a long period of time without monitoring by your doctor.

Antidepressants, used in low doses at bedtime, seem to reduce the effect of some brain chemicals that stimulate the body, producing bruxism and interfering with sleep.

Another medication that helps control pain and inflammation is Toradol. This is a new drug which is very effective and has few side effects. Still another antiinflammatory drug is Naprosyn. This and other medications are usually taken only when pain is severe or at the beginning of TMJ treatment.

In addition to pain medication, skeletal muscle relaxants may be prescribed. I have found that Skelaxin is very effective in reducing muscle pain without the normal side effects of drowsiness. In addition, this medication also contains acetaminophen to help reduce pain.

Parafon Forte DSC is another good muscle relaxant which does not seem to cause as much drowsiness as the well-known, but effective, relaxant Flexeril. However, be aware that Parafon Forte DSC (chlorzoxazone) occasionally causes liver toxicity. If you are taking this drug and develop fever, rash, nausea or vomiting, fatigue, dark urine, yellowing of your skin or of the conjunctiva (white part of your eye), you should notify your doctor immediately. It is also a good idea to avoid drinking alcohol while using this medication.

Antidepressant drugs are also used at times. Remember our discussion about bruxism? Antidepressants, used in low doses at bedtime, seem to reduce the effect of some brain chemicals that stimulate the body, producing bruxism and interfering with sleep.

One such medication is amitriptyline (Elavil). The main side effects are drowsiness, dry mouth and water retention. A second common antidepressant, used for women who suffer with TMJ, is Desyrel. Again, the chief side effect is drowsiness. However, they are very effective in improving sleep and decreasing bruxism.

Although diazepam (Valium) has received bad publicity in recent years, this medication, too, is very effective when used in small doses. Diazepam relaxes muscles (reduces muscle tension) and relieves anxiety, two common complaints of many TMJ sufferers. Drowsiness is the main problem with diazepam. Addiction, when diazepam is used for a long time, may occur as well.

Local anesthetic injections. The use of local anesthetic (novocaine-like medications) injections has been recommended for years to treat muscle pain. Dr. Janet Travell, President Kennedy's personal physician, demonstrated that skeletal muscles develop painful areas termed trigger points. These areas of hypersensitivity in muscles produce predictable pain patterns.

Muscles that move the jaws and those that support the head and neck frequently develop trigger points. These tender areas are usually painful and produce pain at distant sites from the trigger points. This referred pain can be confusing to both doctor and patient.

Trigger points may be felt quite easily. They feel like a small, movable bump under the skin. If compressed, the trigger point will be painful. If compressed firmly and directly, the trigger point will refer pain to a distant site, not necessarily in the same muscle.

These trigger points are treated many different ways. The injection (with a very small needle!) of a small amount of local anesthetic into the trigger point causes muscle relaxation and subsequent reduction or elimination of the referred pain. These trigger points can also be treated by acupressure (hand or finger compression of the trigger points), chiropractic, physical and massotherapy, muscle relaxation, exercise, stress reduction, and dietary changes.

It is important to know that these trigger points can recur, especially after trauma, over-activity, or when you're under stress. The pain produced by this muscle condition is often confused with migraine pain, cervical disc problems, or fibromyalgia (myofibrositis). An accurate diagnosis is a must concerning this disorder. This is a condition that your doctor may choose to refer you for consultation or treatment.

Phase II therapy may include adjustment of the dental occlusion, orthodontics, reconstruction of the teeth, or surgery. Phase II therapy should not be attempted without successful Phase I therapy modalities.

Injection of other medications. In addition to local anesthetics, other medications are injected for specific disorders. For example, injury to a ligament termed the stylomandibular ligament is primarily treated with the injection of an antiinflammatory medication such as cortisone or Sarapin (a nonsteroidal medication). Also, medications may be injected directly into the TMJ for diagnostic purposes or treatment.

Not all dentists perform anesthetic and medication injections. However, these therapies are very important in treating the terrible pain and disorders that accompany TMJ.

Acupuncture. Late in 1997, the National Institutes of Health released a consensus statement supporting the use of acupuncture as part of a comprehensive treatment plan for some conditions. According to the statement, there is some evidence of efficacy in relieving the pain of fibromyalgia, postoperative pain, myofascial pain, and osteoarthritis. Some researchers specifically recommend acupuncture for the facial pain of trigeminal neuralgia and of TMJ dysfunction. This modality is more successful when the cause of pain is neuromuscular rather than due to occlusion or joint damage.

The NIH panel pointed out that acupuncture is associated with a lower risk of adverse events than those associated with drugs or other medical interventions. However, you should be aware that improperly handled or inadequately sterilized acupuncture needles can cause abscesses or septicemia and can spread infection (hepatitis, HIV, subacute bacterial endocarditis).

No patient, under any circumstances, should allow a dentist to perform a complete (full-mouth) adjustment of their teeth without first having all of their symptoms eliminated by conservative treatment modalities.

State regulations for acupuncturists range from stringent to nonexistent. To find a qualified practitioner, consult your state licensing agencies, local medical schools and hospitals, or your doctor. The National Certification Commission of Acupuncture and Oriental Medicine in Washington, DC, can tell you who in your area is qualified; their phone number is (202) 232-1404.

Phase II Therapy

By the time Phase II therapy is begun (except surgery), the patient should be experiencing few if any symptoms. If relief can't be achieved with Phase I therapy, then proceeding to Phase II will only waste time and money. Also, if Phase I therapy has not been successful, then perhaps there is a different physical problem that has not been diagnosed.

Adjustment of the dental occlusion. In recent years, dentists treated TMJ problems by adjusting the occlusion (bite) in an attempt to even the teeth as they touched. However, many teeth were unnecessarily adjusted, mutilated, and some patients saw no improvement but became worse. However, there were many cases in which patients were helped by adjustment of their occlusion when this nonreversible procedure was performed properly.

Current research is showing that TMJ problems may have no connection to dental occlusion and therefore, adjustment of the bite would not be helpful. Again, I can say as a dentist that I have seen many helped and many harmed with occlusal adjustment.

I have seen many patients benefit from surgery when no other mode of treatment helped. However, surgery must be considered with extreme caution; only after all conservative treatments have been tried should surgery be discussed.

Often patients will experience very sensitive teeth, especially to cold. They may be undergoing increased stress in their private or professional life (or both). After a thorough dental examination in which no dental problem can be found (for example, decay or fracture of a tooth), minor occlusal adjustment may very well help reduce the symptoms.

However, no patient, under any circumstances, should allow a dentist to perform a full-mouth adjustment of their teeth without first having all of their symptoms eliminated by conservative treatment modalities (such as splint therapy). This procedure, if performed improperly, can produce terrible TMJ problems which may never be corrected.

Orthodontic treatment. Often, after elimination of TMJ symptoms by using splints or other treatments, the patient and doctor are left with a dilemma: The patient is only comfortable with the splint in his or her mouth; removal of this appliance allows TMJ symptoms to return. In such cases, orthodontic treatment (braces) may be recommended.

However, just as with occlusal adjustment, do not allow anyone, no matter how persuasive, to use orthodontic treatment without first stopping most or all symptoms with a splint. This wonderful but nonreversible mode of treatment (orthodontics) should not be considered without first determining the actual cause or causes of the TMJ symptoms.

Reconstruction of the teeth. What if splint therapy has been successful but you can't go without your splint? In many cases you could consider orthodontic treatment. But what if, for many reasons, you did not wish to have braces? Another option might be a full-mouth reconstruction.

This type of Phase II treatment can be very extensive and expensive. However, often it is the only treatment, except for splint therapy, that will provide long-term relief. As with occlusal adjustment and orthodontics, this type of treatment must not be attempted without TMJ symptoms being eliminated first.

Dentures. Phase II reconstruction might also include restoring the dental occlusion using partial and complete dentures. After relief has been obtained with Phase I therapy, building up old dentures, making new dentures, or making a metal frame (just like an acrylic splint) may be recommended.

Surgery. TMJ surgery has been very controversial. Just a few years ago it was often considered the treatment of choice. Recently, we have realized that TMJ surgery should be attempted, in most cases, only as a last resort. Also, as stated above, you and the doctor must decide what both of you will consider as reasonable or satisfactory treatment results even before Phase II therapy begins.

I have seen many patients benefit from surgery when no other mode of treatment helped. However, surgery must be considered with extreme caution; only after all conservative treatments have been tried should surgery be discussed.

As with back surgery, a high percentage of TMJ surgeries are failures. If the doctor screens the patient and performs an extensive pre-surgical work-up followed by proper post-operative therapy, then the chance for a successful result can be greatly improved.

There are several different types of surgical procedures. A couple, arthrocentesis (rinsing the joint with fluid) and arthroscopy, are at times considered conservative therapy. However, these surgical procedures should not be attempted first without consultation with a TMJ (preferably, a non-surgeon) dentist.

In my own clinical practice, I will recommend aggressive TMJ surgery only after the following three criteria are satisfied:

1. First, all conservative treatment was a failure.
2. Second, there has to be a demonstrable physical or structural explanation for the patient's complaints. A physical problem can be seen with an MRI, x-rays, or with dye injections into the joint (arthrograms).
3. Third, patients must be suffering so much that they must take strong pain medication, and their life-style is greatly altered.

This may seem uncaring; however, it is just the opposite. *I do not want to see anyone undergo an extensive, serious surgical procedure unless an actual reason can be given for the need for surgery.*

If the patient satisfies the above criteria, then he or she must pass one more critical test: *One or both of the TMJs have to be made pain-free with the injection of local anesthetic.* If the pain can't be reduced with anesthetic, then it is quite probable that there is a secondary problem that has yet to be diagnosed, regardless of the results of MRIs or x-rays.

Risks of aggressive surgery must be considered. First and foremost, undergoing surgery does not guarantee elimination of all symptoms. Quite the contrary, you may exchange one set of symptoms for another. Also, the facial nerve can be damaged, resulting in temporary or permanent paralysis of certain facial muscles, including the eyelids. Third, if the patient is not committed to aggressive post-operative treatment and a change in his stress levels, then any surgical procedure will be doomed to failure.

Last of all, if a TMJ sufferer is experiencing severe emotional and/or psychological problems, failure to address these issues will virtually guarantee a surgical failure. Psychological (as well as physical) issues must be considered as sources of unresolved pain complaints.

Six

Disorders that Mimic TMJ

Head and facial pain may be caused by numerous problems, TMJ being only one. Many structures in the head, face and neck areas, when injured, refer pain in and around the TMJ. This often confuses both the patient and the doctors.

Unfortunately, this confusion may lead to inappropriate treatment that may make the patient's pain worse. That is the primary reason why an accurate diagnosis is so important. If the doctor really does not know what the problem is, then he or she will simply take a "shotgun" approach to treatment. All kinds of medication and therapy will be attempted, and as a final resort, surgery will be recommended.

Because of research conducted by committed scientists and clinicians around the world, many pain disorders have been discovered in the past 15 years.

Because of research conducted by committed scientists and clinicians around the world, many pain disorders have been discovered in the past 15 years. Many of these disorders still aren't taught widely in dental or medical school. If the professors themselves haven't learned of these disorders, how can they teach them? So understand that the confusion surrounding TMJ and other such disorders arises from doctors' lack of training. But realize also that we are making progress both in recognizing the significance of these disorders and how to treat them.

Before we proceed, we must distinguish between *disorder* and *disease.* A disease is a pathological process that exhibits classic symptoms. For example, if I mentioned "flu" or "a cold," you would immediately know what I meant. Each of these viral infections have a specific set of symptoms (flu for example: fever, chills, muscle ache, nausea, etc.). Disorders (syndromes), on the other hand, aren't so consistent.

Temporal tendinitis has been the cause of many unnecessary TMJ surgeries. It is diagnosed with an anesthetic injection into the temporal tendon. If symptoms subside after the injection, then you can be reasonably sure that the diagnosis is temporal tendinitis.

Once again, it is important to emphasize that the term "TMJ" is really not accurate; it is used for what the medical community considers as several similar but yet different disorders. These disorders, which may mimic a TMJ problem, have little anatomical connection with the TMJ other than referring pain into and around the joints.

Some of the more common syndromes or pain disorders are: temporal tendinitis, Ernest syndrome, Eagle's syndrome, occipital neuralgia, hyoid bone syndrome, trigeminal neuralgia, and NICO.

Temporal Tendinitis

Temporal tendinitis has been called "The Migraine Mimic" because so many symptoms are similar to migraine headache pain. This condition was first described in 1983, by my mentor and dear friend, Dr. Edwin Ernest. The temporal tendon, a structure which attaches the temporalis muscle to the mandible (Fig. 2), produces approximately six specific referred pain patterns when injured.

As one of the major jaw closing muscles, the temporalis muscle and its tendon may be injured by trauma to the jaw, opening the mouth too wide, severe bruxism, or by building up the bite of the back teeth. Also, a displaced disc of the TMJ can cause the temporalis muscle to contract abnormally putting a great strain on the tendon. If this strain continues over a long period of time, a "tennis elbow" of the jaw can occur, producing severe TMJ-like pain. This pain may be worse with chewing and especially with wide opening of the mouth.

Table 2 lists the common referred pain from an injured temporal tendon. Do you notice anything familiar? Aren't the symptoms similar to TMJ symptoms? That's one major reason why temporal tendinitis and TMJ are so often confused.

Table 2. Symptoms of temporal tendinitis

TMJ Pain
Ear Pain & Pressure
Tooth Sensitivity
Cheek Pain
Eye Pain
Temporal Headache
Neck/Shoulder Pain

This disorder has caused many unnecessary TMJ surgeries. Often, a patient will be treated in a conservative fashion with a splint, medication and physical therapy. If the patient does not respond, then he or she is referred to an oral surgeon. This doctor, seeing that Phase I therapy was not helpful, often performs some type of TMJ surgery. Although the doctors were trying to do their best, the diagnosis and proper treatment of temporal tendinitis was never considered.

But how is temporal tendinitis diagnosed? First, sufferers of temporal tendinitis will have reported many or all of the symptoms listed in Table 2. The real symptom that should alert the doctor is stuffiness and/ or a clogged feeling in the ear. Lastly, the diagnosis is really confirmed after giving a diagnostic anesthetic injection into the temporal tendon. If the pain and other symptoms subside after the injection, then both you and your doctor can be reasonably sure that the diagnosis is temporal tendinitis.

Unfortunately, temporal tendinitis often reoccurs, especially if a person is under a lot of stress, and may require the patient to return for treatment once a year or so.

The treatment of temporal tendinitis is similar to the treatment of tendinitis of any other area of the body. Usually, after the tendon is numb from the local anesthetic injection and if the pain complaints have subsided, then medication is injected into the tendon. The medication used most often is cortisone; however, Sarapin, a nonsteroidal antiinflammatory drug, is used as well. In addition, physical therapy may be recommended. This type of treatment, in conjunction with injections, is quite effective. Also, the use of moist heat over the temple several times per day helps the healing process. If the patient bruxes at night, the doctor might advise that an anti-bruxism splint be made.

If conservative treatment is not successful, then there are two or three surgical procedures for this problem. However, as with TMJ surgery, these invasive approaches should be used only as a last resort.

Unfortunately, temporal tendinitis often reoccurs, especially if a person is under a lot of stress and if he or she is a bruxer or clencher. Understanding this, the patient may have to return for treatment once a year or so. However, at least he or she will have some idea as to the cause of their pain, and time and money won't be wasted looking for relief.

Ernest Syndrome

Ernest Syndrome, named after my mentor and friend, Dr. Edwin Ernest, was first described in the medical literature in the early 1980s. This TMJ-like problem involves the stylomandibular ligament, a tiny structure that connects the base of the skull with the mandibular, or lower jaw (Figure 12). If injured, this structure can produce pain in as many as seven specific regions of the face, head and neck (Table 2).

The stylomandibular ligament prevents the lower jaw from moving too far forward and possibly opening too wide. The ligament tightens when the lower jaw moves forward. Table 3 lists the areas to which the pain of Ernest syndrome is referred.

Table 3. Ernest syndrome: sites of referred pain

The temple
The TMJ
The ear
The cheek
The eye
The throat, especially when swallowing
The lower back teeth and jaw bone

Just like temporal tendinitis, Ernest syndrome's symptoms are frequently confused with symptoms of an injured TMJ.

The most common cause of Ernest syndrome is trauma to the lower jaw. This painful condition may not be noticed for several weeks or months after the injury (which is very common of soft tissue injuries). The best test to see if the stylomandibular ligament is causing pain is to inject a small amount of anesthetic at the attachment of the this structure to the lower jaw.

If the pain subsides after the anesthetic injection, then the ligament is probably the source.

Treatment for Ernest syndrome consists of repeated anesthetic injections followed by cortisone or Sarapin injections into the ligament's attachment to the mandible. Also, anti-inflammatory medications, moist heat, rest and a soft diet are normally recommended. This conservative therapy reduces or eliminates the symptoms of Ernest syndrome about 80% of the time. In those that don't respond to conservative therapy, surgical management is recommended.

Only in the last couple of years has Ernest syndrome been accepted by both the medical and dental communities. Many insurance companies still don't recognize this disorder.

A personal note. I was fortunate, first to have been trained by Dr. Ernest and second, because I was the researcher who conducted and published the first scientific studies concerning Ernest syndrome. Prior to that time (1986), far too many patients received inappropriate treatment and were misdiagnosed for Eagle's syndrome (see below), internal derangements of the TMJ, wisdom tooth problems, and trigeminal neuralgia. These unfortunate persons didn't suffer at the hands of negligent doctors whose only interest was in making money. Not at all.

Only in the last couple of years has Ernest syndrome been accepted by both the medical and dental communities. Many insurance companies still don't recognize this disorder (I can't imagine that!). I have no doubt that my relationship with Dr. Ernest was arranged by Providence.

Eagle's Syndrome

In contrast to Ernest syndrome, the malady most often associated with pharyngeal pain and the styloid process is Eagle's syndrome. This disorder was first fully described by Dr. Watt Eagle in the 1930s. Unfortunately, most doctors, regardless of their degree, confuse this syndrome with Ernest syndrome.

Dr. Eagle advanced the concept that an elongated styloid process (Figure 12) or calcified stylohyoid ligament might cause severe pain and other throat symptoms.

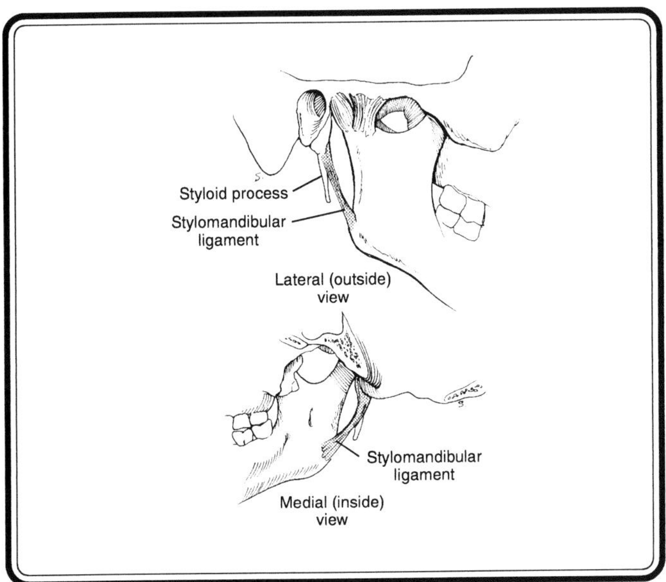

Figure 12. The stylomandibular ligament

Eagle's patients fell into two categories:

1. Those who had the symptoms of a foreign body lodged in the throat, and

2. Those who had neck pain along the distribution of the carotid artery, usually the external branch.

The stylohyoid ligament originates from the tip of the styloid process of the temporal bone and ends by attaching to an area on the hyoid bone, a very small bone in the front part of the throat. The styloid process lies between the internal and external carotid arteries and just behind the back of the throat in the area of the tonsils.

The symptoms of Eagle's syndrome include those shown in Table 4.

Table 4. Symptoms of Eagle's syndrome

1. **A constant dull throat ache** which may be sharp and stabbing, especially when swallowing or turning the head.
2. **Ear pain.** This pain is usually deep and may even feel like an itch. The ear pain is dull but it may be sharp at times.
3. **Difficulty with swallowing.** Often, if the styloid process is elongated or the ligament which runs to the hyoid bone is calcified, swallowing may be irritating or even painful. Many times, patients will complain of the feeling of a chicken or fish bone caught in their throat. They will have to constantly clear their throats and yet, the feeling of a foreign object remains.
4. **Headache.** Eagle's syndrome often produces a temporal headache that is dull but seems to intensify when chewing.

The diagnosis of Eagle's syndrome is based upon the presence of the symptoms listed above, palpation of a tender styloid process, and an elongated styloid process when an x-ray is taken.

Radiologic visualization of an elongated styloid process is very important. The normal styloid process is usually visible with a panoramic x-ray, the one your dentist takes to examine your jaw bones and wisdom teeth.

However, just because the styloid process is elongated doesn't mean that the diagnosis is Eagle's syndrome. In one scientific study of 1771 panoramic x-rays, the researchers reported approximately 18.2% of the radiographs showed varying degrees of elongation of the styloid processes. However, there were no statistical correlations between increasing mineralization, age, and symptoms.

To properly diagnosis Eagle's syndrome, I recommend that a local diagnostic anesthetic injection be given in the area of the tonsils near the styloid process tip. This injection, which may be given either inside or outside of the mouth, is somewhat complicated due to the vital deep structures of the neck in the vicinity of the styloid process tip. The injection may be necessary when Ernest syndrome, myofascial pain dysfunction of the posterior belly of the digastric muscle, or hyoid bone syndrome (discussed below) are also possible diagnoses.

The only treatment for Eagle's syndrome is surgical resection of the styloid process and/or the ossified stylohyoid ligament. Surgery is usually simple and may be performed either in the throat or from the outside, depending upon the surgeon's training. Usually, ENT doctors operate from the outside and oral surgeons from the inside of the throat.

Hyoid Bone Syndrome

In 1954, Dr. L.A. Brown reported a pain syndrome that he identified as the hyoid bone syndrome. This rather obscure pain disorder produces chronic or recurrent pain in the area of the side of the neck near the hyoid bone.

The hyoid bone is a U-shaped structure that lies in the front of the neck above the larynx (Adam's apple). It is the only bone of the body that does not articulate with any other bone. Attaching to it are several muscles and ligaments, permitting it to stabilize the head as you swallow. In fact, you can feel the hyoid bone. It's about one finger's breadth above the Adam's apple. If you swallow while your finger is in place, you'll be able to feel the bone move up and down slightly.

Symptoms of hyoid bone syndrome include those listed in Table 5.

Table 5. Symptoms of hyoid bone syndrome

1. Chronic, constant pain in the lateral side of the throat. The pain, which can be either sharp or dull, radiates to the ear, throat, temple, cheek, TMJ, sternocleidomastoid muscle, and the back of the throat.
2. Pain in the lower molar teeth which may make you think that you have a cavity.
3. Upper chest pain which may extend down to the level of the middle of the breast without extending below the nipple.
4. Dizziness or even fainting when turning the head towards the injured side.
5. Pain when swallowing.
6. A chronic sore throat and at times, difficulty or tightness when swallowing.
7. At times, like Eagle's syndrome, some people report the sensation of a foreign body in the throat with dull pain when swallowing.

The establishment of an accurate diagnosis of hyoid bone syndrome, as with other pain syndromes, requires both a careful gathering of the history and a meticulous physical examination. The most common cause of hyoid bone syndrome is trauma. The patients I've found with this disorder have either hit their throats on the steering wheel in an accident, have experienced violent vomiting, or have been strangled.

Diagnostic testing for hyoid bone syndrome is best performed by giving a diagnostic anaesthetic injection. Unfortunately, unless the portions of the hyoid bone are out of place, a fracture in the small bone is very difficult to see on an x-ray or other imaging tests.

Various types of conservative, non-surgical treatment have been attempted in the treatment of hyoid bone syndrome. These include physical therapy, infiltration of local anaesthetic with cortisone, and oral cortisone.

However, the only predictable and successful treatment that I've found is surgery of the fractured area of the hyoid bone. Actually, the procedure is quite simple and can even be performed as an outpatient or office procedure with local anaesthetic in most cases.

Patients with hyoid bone syndrome have either hit their throats on the steering wheel in an accident, have experienced violent vomiting, or have been strangled. Surgical treatment is a simple procedure performed on an outpatient basis.

Occipital Neuralgia

Occipital neuralgia is generally ignored in the medical textbooks. This disorder is characterized by pain located in the cervical and posterior regions of the head (these are the occipital areas) which may or may not extend or radiate into the sides of the head and ultimately, into the facial and frontal regions.

There are three subcategories of occipital neuralgia, two of which we'll discuss here: lesser occipital nerve neuralgia and greater occipital nerve neuralgia. The third, myofascial pain dysfunction syndrome, is presented in depth in Chapter 9. All three of these are often misdiagnosed as fibromyalgia (myofibrositis or fibrositis) or worse, cervical spine arthritis or a cervical disc problem. Occipital pain also commonly occurs with TMJ, often magnifying the pain in the face and temples that is primarily caused by TMJ.

Occipital neuralgia often occurs after a whiplash injury, a blow to the back of the head, or an injury that produces a twisting of the head.

The pain symptoms of occipital neuralgia occur quite often in persons who must sit at a keyboard or typewriter for a long time and in persons who must bend or tilt their heads for any length of time (such as painters, factory workers and construction workers). Also, these symptoms might occur while sitting for a long time looking up at a speaker or a movie.

Occipital neuralgia occurs often in persons who must sit for long hours at a computer and in those who bend or tilt their heads for any length of time (painters, factory workers and construction workers). These symptoms might also occur while sitting for a long time looking up at a speaker or a movie.

Lesser Occipital Nerve Neuralgia is the most common cervical nerve disorder. I can attest to this statement based upon over 19 years of clinical experience. This disorder is most frequently seen after trauma such as extension-flexion (whiplash) injuries arising from a motor vehicle accident or striking the back of the head during a fall.

A common cause of lesser occipital nerve neuralgia is iatrogenic trauma while under the influence of a general anaesthetic. During a surgical procedure, the patient's head oftentimes must be rotated or the neck extended. Again, symptoms may develop immediately after the procedure, but more commonly they don't appear for a few days to weeks.

Patients may wander from physical therapist to chiropractor to medical doctor to dentist. They may be treated with muscle relaxants, antiinflammatory analgesics and even blood pressure medication. Unfortunately, the medications rarely provide any lasting relief. These patients are frequently scorned as malingerers by attorneys and physicians alike.

Also known as the minor occipital nerve, the lesser occipital nerve varies in size and is sometimes double. It arises from portions of the 2nd and 3rd cervical nerves. The lesser occipital nerve courses over the middle scalene muscle, winds around the posterior border of the sternocleidomastoid muscle and near the base of the skull. It then sends branches up the back of the head in the scalp behind the ear, supplying feeling to the skin of the back of the head and the skin of the ear. It converges with many other nerves, including branches of the trigeminal nerve, the major nerve which supplies feeling to the superficial and deep structures of the face, mouth, and TMJ.

The symptoms of lesser occipital nerve neuralgia are listed in Table 6.

Table 6. Symptoms of lesser occipital nerve neuralgia

1. Occipital pain which may effect both sides of the back of the head.
2. Pain radiation from the back of the head to the sides and temples, cheeks and even the forehead.
3. Pain and/or pressure behind the eye.
4. Light sensitivity. Sufferers often wear sunglasses even on cloudy days.
5. Nausea when the pain is severe.
6. Pain radiation into the ear, shoulder and at times, the arm.

If you suffer with lesser occipital nerve neuralgia, you'll notice pain that is dull and constant. The pain will vary in intensity depending on your physical activities and emotional stress. You might experience minimal pain relief from muscle relaxants and antiinflammatory medications; but, generally, the pain will persist no matter what you do. Often, physical therapy or chiropractic treatment will help for a short period of time, and then the pain will return.

The diagnosis of lesser occipital nerve neuralgia is best proven by the effective use of a diagnostic anaesthetic injection of the lesser occipital nerve.

Fortunately, conservative treatment tends to succeed even for chronic cases of occipital neuralgia. As always, attempt all non-surgical types of treatment before you even consider surgery, and if you have any doubt, demand a second or even third opinion.

Fortunately, conservative treatment tends to be quite successful even for chronic cases. Medicine is injected, along with a long-lasting local anesthetic, into the back of the head around the lesser occipital nerve. I instruct patients to use ice over the painful area and I often prescribe a muscle relaxant and an antiinflammatory medication. Patients shouldn't lift anything weighing more than 10 pounds for several days. Moist heat can be used over the painful neck area several times per day. Treatment by a chiropractor, medical massage therapist, or physical therapist is helpful in conjunction with the injections and medication. The injections usually have to be repeated a few times.

Surgical treatment is needed about 40% of the time, and several types of procedures may be used.

Greater occipital nerve neuralgia. As with lesser occipital neuralgia, greater occipital nerve neuralgia is one of the two and perhaps three different disorders referred to collectively in most literature as occipital neuralgia.

The greater occipital nerve is a branch of the second cervical nerve. It runs up the back of the head and supplies feeling to the skin of the scalp as far forward as the top of the skull.

The symptoms of greater occipital nerve neuralgia are similar but yet distinctly different from those of lesser occipital nerve neuralgia. They include those listed in Table 7.

Table 7. Symptoms of greater occipital neuralgia

1. Occipital pain that radiates to the top of the head. This pain is usually constant, dull, and varies in intensity. When severe, the pain is throbbing, sometimes with shock-like jabs. The sufferer is often awakened at night with pain and generally has pain upon waking.
2. Pain in the temple which may be confused for a muscle contraction headache.
3. Pain above and around the eye, especially on the outer side.
4. At time, pain radiation into the lateral side of the jaw.
5. Dizziness which is worsened by both physical activity and emotional stress.

Trauma seems to be the main cause of this disorder, but there is also some evidence that a displaced disc in the TMJ may also be a cause. Also, cervical degenerative arthritis and sitting in one position repeatedly for prolonged periods of time may be causes.

As with many other pain syndromes, the diagnosis of greater occipital nerve neuralgia is primarily based upon the success of an anaesthetic block of the greater occipital nerve.

Treatment of greater occipital nerve neuralgia is virtually the same as for the lesser form. Fortunately, physical therapy is very effective in reducing the symptoms. Since the pain is often present when waking, I often prescribe a tricyclic antidepressant (for example, amitriptyline 10 to 25 mg) or Ambien 5 mg at night to improve sleep. These medications are very helpful for all types of chronic pain conditions. Natural remedies are also very helpful (see Chapter 13).

Lastly, surgery may be needed if conservative therapy fails. However, as always, attempt all non-surgical types of treatment before you even consider surgery, and if you have any doubt, demand a second or even third opinion.

Trigeminal Neuralgia

Trigeminal neuralgia is a terrible disorder of the trigeminal, or fifth cranial nerve. This is one of the most painful problems that plagues human beings. In fact, its description first appeared in the scientific literature in 1672 under the name *tic douloureux*, which in French literally means unbearably painful twitch. Far too often, when a person is suffering with severe facial pain with no apparent cause, the diagnosis given is trigeminal neuralgia. Because of this, the patient may be subjected to medications and even very serious surgical procedures that are not necessary.

The trigeminal nerve is the largest and most influential (in area) cranial nerve. (Cranial nerves are nerves which come directly off the brain.) There are three large divisions of this nerve. In turn, these divisions divide into smaller branches that supply the face, eyes, TMJs, mouth, nose, teeth, palate, the throat, and the muscles of mastication.

Trigeminal neuralgia can actually be divided into three distinct disorders:

1. Typical trigeminal neuralgia
2. Atypical trigeminal neuralgia
3. Atypical facial pain

These three disorders are frequently confused.

Typical trigeminal neuralgia, which is known classically as *tic douloureux*, usually afflicts persons in their fifties or older. It is caused by compression of the nerve inside the skull by a tiny blood vessel or even by a tumor. Six percent or so of those with the typical type also have multiple sclerosis.

The symptoms of tic douloureux (Table 8) are quite characteristic and specific.

Table 8. Symptoms of typical trigeminal neuralgia

1. Sharp electrical pain that lasts for seconds.
2. Pain is triggered by touching a specific area of the skin by washing, shaving, applying makeup, brushing the teeth, kissing, or even cold air.
3. The second division of the trigeminal nerve (the maxillary division), which supplies feeling to the mid-face, upper teeth and palate, seems to be involved most.
4. The pain is so severe that the sufferer will do virtually anything to avoid touching the trigger zone and producing the pain.

Treatment of typical trigeminal neuralgia is primarily with medication. For years, the drug Tegretol has been used for treatment. Unfortunately, this drug has serious side effects, the chief one being damage to the cells that produce blood cells. Drowsiness is also a common problem with Tegretol.

A newer medication, Baclofen, has been a wonderful drug for the treatment of trigeminal neuralgia. Although Baclofen also has the potential to cause drowsiness, this side effect is usually not as severe as with Tegretol.

Recently, we've been using new medication, Neurontin, alone and with Baclofen for the treatment of trigeminal neuralgia with excellent success.

If treatment with medications does not adequately control the pain, then treatment of individual branches of the trigeminal nerve is attempted. Local anesthetic injections with cortisone may be helpful. If not, then some neurosurgeons inject alcohol or glycerin directly into sections of the nerve. The intent is to actually damage the nerve to produce a long-lasting anesthesia. This procedure, when successful, usually needs to be repeated.

If all else fails, brain surgery needs to be considered. This decision would be made by a neurosurgeon. One of several different surgical procedures may be recommended.

Atypical trigeminal neuralgia. In contrast to the typical type, atypical trigeminal neuralgia seems to cause pain constantly with the intensity increasing and decreasing. There are trigger zones with this type; however, there also is an area of dull aching that is intensified by touching the trigger zones. All three divisions of the trigeminal nerve seems to be affected equally. A common cause of this disorder is trauma, especially after a surgical incision or blow to the face.

Diagnosis of atypical trigeminal neuralgia is made by ruling out other problems (for example, an abscessed tooth). To determine specifically which part of the trigeminal nerve is producing pain, a diagnostic anesthetic injection is used to eliminate the pain.

We treat this disorder by injecting an antiinflammatory medication and prescribing Baclofen, Neurontin, or both. These injections may have to be repeated several times. If this conservative therapy is not successful, then surgery must be considered.

Atypical facial pain. Atypical facial pain is a disorder that also affects the trigeminal nerve. However, the symptoms are not clearly defined as they are in typical and atypical trigeminal neuralgia. Atypical facial pain seems to affect people who are under a tremendous amount of stress and may even have a history of psychiatric problems. This does not mean that if you suffer with atypical facial pain that you're mentally ill. Rather, since there's no absolute, diagnostic test for atypical facial pain, many symptoms and types of patients get thrown into this nebulous category.

In my practice, I've not found but two or three patients with this problem who also needed psychological counseling. Even then, I had to wonder if that was because no one believed their complaint of facial pain. Also, as with most of us in today's fast-paced society, stress is a major factor in our lives. Unfortunately, those with facial pain seemed to be affected more by stress. Therefore, if doctors can't find the cause for a pain disorder and the patient is in the midst of stress (who isn't?), then it is assumed that there is a psychological cause for the undiagnosed pain.

Table 9: Comparison of symptoms of trigeminal neuralgia (typical and atypical) and atypical facial pain

	Typical TGN	**Atypical TGN**	**Atypical Facial Pain**
Character of Pain	Sharp, Electrical	Dull	Varies
Duration	Seconds	Constant	Constant
Frequency	Intermittent	Constant	Constant
Location	V2* & V3+	All 3 Divisions	Vague
Triggers	Extra-Oral	Varies	Vague
Stress Induced	No	No	Possibly

*V2: Maxillary division of the trigeminal nerve

+V3: Mandibular division of the trigeminal nerve

Treatment for atypical facial pain must be directed towards elimination of the symptoms. Medications, anesthetic injections and stress management are helpful at times. Surgery should definitely not be considered unless a specific structure that is producing the pain can be isolated.

A True Story

In my practice, I've not found but 2 or 3 patients with atypical facial pain who also needed psychological counseling. Even then, I wondered if that was because no one believed their complaint of facial pain.

I'd like to introduce you to Dorothy W. Her story is typical and should be told at this time. Dorothy, who was living in a distant state, was referred to our office for evaluation of left trigeminal neuralgia. She was 65 years old, her husband was 72. He had retired from a public utility company five years earlier, just about the time that her pain began. They had spent more than $35,000 of their retirement money, had seen numerous doctors, and she had undergone three neurosurgical procedures. All attempts to relieve her pain had failed.

Her plight reminded me of the woman with chronic bleeding in the book of Mark (5:24-34). She, too, had suffered for years, spent all her money, and was worse, not better.

When I interviewed Dorothy, she was discouraged and fearful. She told me that she was suffering with left facial pain which started in the lower jaw and started like a jab or a bolt of lightening, producing left ear and temple pain. She couldn't chew, talk, sing at church, or even kiss her husband without experiencing this intense pain.

Do her symptoms sound familiar? Are you thinking trigeminal neuralgia? Then you're not alone. So were the previous doctors. She'd been treated by at least four of them! In addition to all types of medication, Dorothy had also undergone three neurosurgical procedures, which didn't help and only made her worse!

Knowing at least one previous and very prominent doctor, I felt that there must have been something causing her pain other than trigeminal neuralgia. I asked her one simple question: "Does your left TMJ click or did it used to click?" Her answer was a resounding, "Yes!" Immediately, I examined her TMJs. Pushing on the lower jaw produced the pain. I injected the left joint with local anesthetic and within five minutes, all symptoms had subsided. Her diagnosis: a displaced articular disc in the left TMJ, not trigeminal neuralgia.

I initially treated Dorothy with a splint and she did great—no further pain. Phase II Therapy simply consisted of making a metal splint and today, more than 17 years later, she is still pain free.

Neuralgia-Inducing Cavitational Osteonecrosis (NICO)

As recently as 1979, a newly described pain disorder was reported by two separate researchers. This disorder, called osteocavitational lesions or Ratner's bone cavities, produced pain similar to that of trigeminal neuralgia. In fact, trigeminal neuralgia was the diagnosis usually received by these patients.

In 1992, oral pathologist Dr. Jerry Bouquot wrote a paper that was instrumental in changing the name to *Neuralgia-Inducing Cavitational Osteonecrosis* (NICO). In plain English(!), this means pain due to dead bone.

For years, orthopedic surgeons have been challenged with the problem of bone death in the head of the femur (ball portion of the upper leg bone). It now appears that bone death can also occur in the jaws, especially the mandible.

NICO appears to develop in the same way as bone death in the head the femur: blockages in the tiny blood vessels, perhaps by blood clots formed due to a malfunctioning clotting reaction. Apparently, minute blood clots prevent blood flow, which "robs" oxygen from areas of bone. This lack of oxygen, plus chronic bone inflammation due to a dead tooth, an abscessed tooth, or poor healing after surgery, results in bone death and the symptoms of NICO.

Sadly, don't expect most doctors to even know about NICO, since its appearance in the scientific literature has only been recent.

Diagnosis is complicated by the fact that x-rays are usually normal. Also, NICO produces referred pain patterns that confuse both patient and doctor. Just like trigeminal neuralgia, there are trigger areas that, when pressed, produce pain. These trigger areas develop directly over the areas of dead bone. The mandible is affected more often than the upper jaw.

One important aspect of NICO is a history of tooth extraction, especially lower back teeth, usually years earlier. Small areas of bone actually die, producing neuralgia-like pain symptoms. It appears that after a tooth extraction, NICO may develop due to injury of the blood vessels in the area that ultimately results in poor circulation. This bone infection, called *osteomyelitis,* has been recognized for years in other parts of the body. Yet, in the form of NICO, it is a newly described problem.

The pain referral patterns (Figure 13) are confusing. Pain may be radiated into the face, head, TMJ, neck, shoulder and even the arm. Trigger areas in the mouth, when compressed, reproduce referred pain patterns. Again, the most striking symptom of this disorder is normal x-ray findings.

Even if you point to a trigger area and an x-ray is taken, the bone will appear normal. Understandably, the doctor is likely to abandon his or her search of that area.

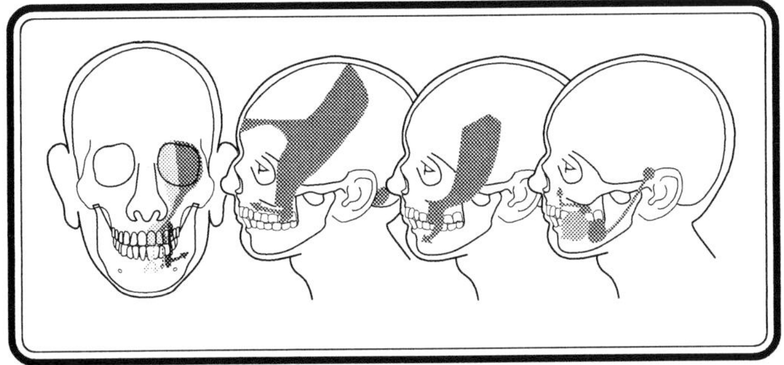

Figure 13. Referred pain patterns of NICO

An accurate diagnosis can be made by using selective local anesthetic injections to "turn-off" the trigger areas in the bone. Once the NICO areas are located (and frequently there are several), they must be treated with surgery.

Again, as with internal TMJ problems, don't allow anyone to recommend surgery for NICO unless he or she can stop the pain with a local anesthetic injection. And sadly, don't expect most doctors to even know of this pain disorder since its appearance in the scientific literature has only been recent.

Summary

In this chapter, we have discussed many pain disorders that mimic a TMJ problem. Do you now realize how difficult and complicated it is to make an accurate diagnosis of one of these? Being syndromes and not actual diseases, frequently they don't exhibit all of the listed symptoms. This further confuses their presentation.

Doctors are trained to listen to symptoms, observe signs, and place these findings into neat packages to determine a diagnosis. Therefore, if several disorders have similar symptoms, their recognition is confused.

What's the answer? Unfortunately, patients, at times, must educate the doctors. If a doctor has no training concerning Ernest syndrome, for example, then he or she will not be familiar with the symptoms and signs of this painful problem or may even confuse it with Eagle's syndrome. This might lead to ineffective treatment or worse yet, inappropriate treatment. However, you, the patient, may have to educate this practitioner and if he is not willing to listen, find another doctor.

Realize that you may not be well received if you immediately charge in and begin lecturing to this learned person. Allow him or her some grace. Everyone can't know everything about everything (this, of course, includes you and me).

However, don't permit the doctor to proceed with any invasive or irreversible procedure until he or she can prove that your problem is understood. Insist on a referral, if necessary. Remember, you may be a patient, but you're also a consumer and, in my opinion, your health care is your responsibility, not any doctor's.

Seven

Muscle Pain

So far, we've discussed TMJ pain and disorders that mimic TMJ. Another category of pain disorders is produced by skeletal muscle pain. All skeletal muscles are capable of producing pain and referring pain when they are not functioning properly. Often, local pain at the site of injury in a skeletal muscle is complicated by the fact that these muscles refer pain away from the painful area, complicating diagnosis.

When it comes to muscle pain syndromes, confusion abounds! The International Association for the Study of Pain classifies chronic muscle pain syndromes "without probable cause" into two categories:

1. Fibromyalgia or myofibrositis
2. Myofascial pain syndrome, also known as myofascial pain dysfunction syndrome (MPDS)

These disorders are similar and yet quite different. Often confused one for the other, both syndromes produce painful muscles and referred pain. Fibromyalgia is generalized throughout the body whereas myofascial pain dysfunction generally refers to the muscles of mastication and the neck and shoulder muscles.

Trauma may be associated with either fibromyalgia or MPDS, injuring muscle tissue, which then develops a trigger point (small area of muscle contraction). Trauma may be as obvious as a car accident or a blow with a fist. Or trauma may be as subtle as over-exertion playing softball at a picnic. Whatever the cause, the effects are the same: muscle pain, referred pain, and muscle dysfunction.

Healthy muscles contract when active and relax when inactive. Injury or chronic stress can cause prolonged muscle contraction. After a time, the muscles go into spasm, unable to relax. Painful chemicals like lactic acid accumulate, robbing the muscles of valuable oxygen. This in turn perpetuates the muscle contraction, thus forming a trigger point.

Healthy muscles contract when active and relax when inactive. Injury or chronic stress can cause prolonged muscle contraction. After a time, the muscles go into spasm, unable to relax.

This condition produces a reflex through the spinal cord, causing more muscle spasm and chemical build-up, and continues until the reflex is interrupted, allowing the muscle to relax. Exercise might stop the spasm; however, with a severe injury, normal exercise may not be possible.

As the trigger point remains, it then refers pain to distant sites, confusing the sufferer and any doctor attempting to perform an examination. Trigger points may remain for an indefinite length of time, even years. These areas of muscle contraction produce muscle dysfunction (restricted activity and efficiency). In the neck, for example, this will be noticed as a limitation of movement of the head in certain directions; in the jaw, a limitation of opening of the mouth.

Whether the problem is myofascial pain or the much broader fibromyalgia, pain and dysfunction are exacerbated by many of the same factors: trauma, chilling, over-use, or being in a position for a prolonged period of time.

Fibromyalgia

Fibromyalgia is a chronic, painful muscle condition characterized by painful skeletal muscles and other soft tissue throughout the body.

Although Hippocrates first described fibromyalgia, only in the last few years has the medical community paid much attention (and given credence) to this syndrome. The controversy and disbelief associated with fibromyalgia arose because this disorder does not present objective evidence in the form of x-rays, biopsies or routine lab tests.

Research about fibromyalgia started to appear in medical journals in the late 1960s. In 1987, an article published in the *Journal of the American Medical Association* validated the existence of fibromyalgia as a legitimate syndrome recognized by the American Medical Association. Fortunately for sufferers, this syndrome is now more widely accepted by many, but not all, doctors.

Although Hippocrates first described fibromyalgia, the medical profession was hard to convince it really existed because objective evidence in the form of x-rays or biopsies couldn't be found.

In people with this disorder, levels of many neurotransmitters and hormones are abnormal. Also, results of thermography (the measurement of heat produced by areas of the body) are substantially different in people with fibromyalgia. However, tests for these abnormalities are specialized and not considered routine. At this time no single laboratory testing procedure exists to diagnose fibromyalgia.

Fibromyalgia is diagnosed based on patient history and clinical examination. The "signature" of fibromyalgia is the presence of specific tender points. Because they have a peculiar, abnormal consistency, tender points are considered objective examination findings that can be detected by an experienced doctor.

Fibromyalgia is characterized by signs and symptoms listed in Table 10.

Table 10. Symptoms of fibromyalgia

1. Generalized muscle soreness and stiffness lasting more than three months
2. Poor sleep with morning fatigue and stiffness
3. Tenderness at 11 of 18 specific sites
4. Tingling and/or numbness
5. Swelling
6. Cold intolerance
4. Normal blood test results

The more common painful areas are the low cervical spine, the shoulder, the second rib, the arm, the buttocks and the knee. These symptoms are often worsened by stress or a change in the weather. Physical activity not only increases the patient's pain complaints, but also makes the next few days miserable, producing intense muscle pain.

Depression, which may be due to a chemical imbalance in the brain or the development of chronic pain, is common with fibromyalgia.

Treatment of fibromyalgia includes physical therapy, trigger point anesthetic injections, stress management, nonsteroidal anti-inflammatory drugs, dietary changes and antidepressant drugs, especially at bedtime.

Although many TMJ patients suffer with both fibromyalgia and MPDS, more frequently they're afflicted with MPDS. For further information about fibromyalgia, see Appendix B.

Before we leave the topic of fibromyalgia, I'd like to mention a new type of treatment. Dr. Paul St. Amand discovered by accident that fibromyalgia patients seemed to respond to the use of the common decongestant guaifenesin (pronounced, "gwhy-fen-es-sin").

This medication is commonly used for chest colds as an expectorant, but you can't just take cough medicine to treat fibromyalgia. After talking with Dr. St. Amand, I've been using guaifenesin with excellent results for both fibromyalgia and MPDS patients.

Myofascial Pain Dysfunction Syndrome

Like fibromyalgia, myofascial pain dysfunction syndrome (MPDS) is a painful condition of the skeletal muscles. Usually when we refer to MPDS, we are referring to the muscles of mastication as well as the neck and shoulder muscles. However, this doesn't mean that other skeletal muscles aren't affected, for they may be. But the muscles of mastication and the neck and shoulder muscles seem to be most commonly involved.

MPDS refers to skeletal muscles (*myo* refers to muscle) and their thin membrane (*fascia*) covering. A trigger point in the muscle or the junction of the muscle and fascia (hence, *myofascial pain*) develops due to any number of causes. This trigger point is locally tender and when active, refers pain through specific patterns to distant areas. For example, trigger points in the temporalis muscle may even produce tooth pain, confusing both patient and dentist, often precipitating unnecessary root canal therapy or extraction of healthy teeth.

Trigger points. According to Drs. Travell and Simons, probably the two most knowledgeable people in the world about myofascial pain, trigger points have several characteristics (Table 11).

Table 11. Characteristics of trigger points

1. Myofascial pain is referred away from trigger points in very specific patterns characteristic of each skeletal muscle. Often, we can determine the location of the trigger point just by the way the patient's pain develops.

2. The pain is often dull, aching and deep and may intensify to severe and torturing pain.

3. Latent trigger points (those which are present in the muscle but don't normally cause pain) are activated by over-work, fatigue, direct injury, and chilling (like sitting near an air conditioner).

4. Trigger points vary in pain from time to time and from day to day, depending upon many physical factors as well as stress levels.

5. The symptoms of myofascial trigger points long outlast the cause. Injured muscles, directed by the brain, seem to "learn" new movements in order to avoid activating latent trigger points.

6. Trigger points may cause other problems such as sweating (very common on the skin of the lower back; termed pseudomotor activity), reddening skin, dizziness and even disorientation.

Symptoms of MPDS. Symptoms of MPDS are generally caused by the development of one or many skeletal muscle trigger points. Symptoms may also be caused by hormonal changes (especially in those women who suffer with premenstrual syndrome), biochemical changes alone or in conjunction with chronic pain problems. Also, postural changes due to injuries in other areas of the body (for example, a cast on a broken foot) may produce myofascial pain symptoms. (See Table 12.)

Table 12. Symptoms of myofascial pain dysfunction syndrome

1. A history of growing pains as a child. Believe it or not, many people develop MPDS as a child or young teenager.

2. A history of sudden onset during or shortly after acute stress, physical activity, or muscle fatigue.

3. Dull, aching deep muscular pain that is intensified by pressure on the trigger points within the painful muscles.

4. A reduction of motion of the head (if neck and shoulder muscles are involved) or reduction in jaw movement (if the muscles of mastication are affected).

5. Shooting pains from the neck, often being mistaken as a cervical disc problem.

6. Physical activity such as chewing, lifting or running may aggravate the MPD symptoms, further reducing the motion of the head and jaw.

7. Allergies. Many people seem to have multiple allergies, especially to the common chemical histamine, a very potent vasodilator (causes small blood vessels to open up) which is released from mast cells in the blood. Have you noticed that most allergy medications are some type of antihistamine?

MPDS is frequently confused with migraine, cervical disk degeneration, even pleurisy. In addition to direct trauma and muscle injury, MPDS is caused by over-activity (especially without adequate warm-up and cool-down) and over-exertion. Sitting directly under an air conditioning duct can activate quiescent (latent) trigger points. Also, standing or sitting in one position for a prolonged period of time may cause formation of trigger points, thus producing MPDS. Further, other diseases, such as arthritis and gall bladder problems, may produce MPDS.

Treatment of MPDS. Treatment must be aimed at the elimination of trigger points. This may be with medications (muscle relaxants), moist heat, stretching, or elimination of postural habits. Change positions frequently, whether you're sitting at a computer or riding in a car or plane. Also, get up from your desk and stretch a couple times each hour.

Change positions frequently, whether you're sitting at a computer or riding in a car or plane. Also, get up from your desk and stretch a couple times each hour.

If you plan to engage in a sport or physical activity, first warm up slowly and stretch. Make sure you take your time and be thorough. Stretching and warming up will not only reduce trigger point formation but also reduce the risk of several other kinds of soft tissue injuries.

If you're sleeping in a hotel room, check the direction that the air conditioner blows air. Don't sleep directly under or in the path of chilled air. This also is a good rule when sitting in a car, plane, or when working. Avoid sitting directly under an air conditioner duct. If you can't change your position, cover your neck and shoulders with a light jacket or sweater.

If you're a secretary, a receptionist, an insurance agent, or anyone else who has to spend most of their time on the telephone, purchase a hands-free headset. Use this device instead of trying to cradle the phone between your head and shoulder. Holding the phone for a long time in such an unnatural manner will produce trigger points in the neck and shoulders, especially in air conditioning. Such hands-free telephones are very inexpensive and replace the regular phone's receiver in a matter of seconds.

I once treated a patient with TMJ and MPDS in such a manner. She was the receptionist of a very busy gynecological practice and you can imagine, she was on the phone literally from morning until night. I simply prescribed a hands-free headset and within a week, all her symptoms were gone, and this was more than 10 years ago!

If you spend most of your time on the telephone, use a hands-free headset instead of cradling the phone between your head and shoulder. I once treated a patient with TMJ and MPDS in such a manner. Within a week, all her symptoms were gone, and this was more than 10 years ago!

Many people develop MPDS in the muscles of mastication by grinding and clenching their teeth, especially when they are under a lot of stress. In fact, there may be a decrease in opening of the mouth which might be misdiagnosed as a TMJ disc problem. Chronic clenching of the teeth causes the muscles in the neck and shoulders to become tense, develop trigger points and reduce motion of the head and neck. If this occurs to you, relax!

Try to eliminate some of the stressing factors in your life and adopt a more relaxed attitude. If you continue to clench, see a dentist for the fabrication of a splint. Also, consult a chiropractor or medical massage therapist if neck and shoulder pain persist. Use moist heat over the painful muscles and treat the trigger points with acupressure (see Chapter 11).

Your doctor may prescribe muscle relaxants and antiinflammatory medications for a few weeks. A common way to treat both fibromyalgia and MPDS is by trigger point injections with local anesthetics in conjunction with medications. He or she may even prescribe specific medication to be taken at bedtime. Don't allow anyone to recommend invasive, nonreversible procedures like surgery. Get a second opinion.

To reduce the effects of these muscle disorders, eliminate caffeine from your diet. Caffeine is a naturally occurring chemical found in the leaves, seeds or fruits of more than 60 plants. The most common plants are coffee and cocoa beans, kola nuts, and tea leaves. This chemical is a mild stimulant to the body, especially skeletal muscles. We may drink coffee or tea for stimulation and to make us alert, but it affects everyone differently and can worsen muscle symptoms.

Caffeine does not accumulate in the blood and is excreted from the body within a few hours after consumption. It may produce restlessness, nervousness, excitement, insomnia, frequent urination, muscle twitching, tachycardia (racing heart beat) or cardiac arrhythmia (alteration of heart beats), and agitation. However, caffeine also constricts blood vessels which will further starve the muscles of nutrients and oxygen, thus once again, perpetuating trigger points, pain and referred pain.

Caffeine is used in certain medications, which you should avoid if you suffer with either fibromyalgia or MPDS. Table 13 lists some of the foods, drinks and medications that contain caffeine. Avoid these foods whenever possible, especially if you suffer from fibromyalgia or MPDS.

Common misconceptions about MPDS. MPDS is still not understood or even recognized by many doctors, and perhaps that's because there are so many misconceptions about this common pain syndrome. Fortunately, alternative medicine advocates and proponents are forcing the more traditional medical people to at least listen to patients who complain about the effects of trigger points.

Some of the more common misconceptions of MPDS are listed on the next page.

1. *Since they can't be observed with x-rays, blood tests, or MRI scans (in other words, normal laboratory tests), then myofascial trigger points must be psychogenic, or "all in the head" of the sufferer.* This is a sad point of view. For many years, even Dr. Janet Travell fought against the medical establishment. **Only in the last few years have these concepts been recognized as valid . . . by most.**

2. *Only certain personality types seem to develop MPDS.* Unfortunately, the typical MPDS sufferer is categorized as a young to middle-aged female who is a perfectionist, intense, highly motivated and goal oriented. This is not true. Of course, this personality type sufferers with many chronic problems associated with stress, but so do other personality types. **MPDS knows no personality, sexual or age boundary.**

3. *Trigger points are self-limited and need no treatment.* As a sufferer of MPDS and a doctor who treats this problem, I can state this is also not true. **Trigger points may become quiet, but they are still present as latent trigger points, easily activated by stressors such as fatigue, emotional stress, over-activity or cold breezes.**

4. *MPDS is not severe and therefore, doesn't need to be treated.* Although MPDS is not a life-threatening disorder, it still needs to be treated aggressively and taken seriously. The presence of trigger points make life totally miserable and rob the sufferer of many joys of life. **Why should we ignore MPDS when it can be treated so effectively?**

MPDS has to be taken seriously by doctors and therapists and included in their process of diagnosis. Find a doctor who understands and treats MPDS and fibromyalgia. For fibromyalgia and MPDS, a chiropractor or osteopathic physician may be your doctor of choice. Medical massage therapists can be effective in treating MPDS.

If you also have TMJ symptoms, consider consulting with a dentist who treats TMJ and MPDS. Many sufferers find excellent relief with medical massage therapists, too.

Lastly, consider consulting a naturopathic doctor (an ND), who is a licensed practitioner in many states who primarily uses nutrition and holistic approaches to these and other diseases and disorders. (See Chapter 14 and Appendix B for more information.) Above all, don't allow anyone to perform invasive or surgical procedures until you're sure of the diagnosis and competency of the practitioner. As always, get a second opinion, and if your doctor is offended by such an idea, find a new doctor.

The computer age. Unless you've been living in a cave for the last five years or so, you know that computers have descended on our lives like a summer storm. Hardly a job today doesn't, at times, require the use of a computer. Many people sit for hour upon hour at a computer screen, and they wonder why they have neck, head and shoulder pain.

I've found with many of my patients that simply changing the position of the computer screen so that it is directly in front of you eliminates the development of MPDS trigger points. Also, desks are rarely made for function. Usually, the position of the computer keyboard is too high, thus causing the formation of trigger points in the neck and shoulders.

Make sure that the keyboard is at the proper height. You may need to open the desk drawer and place the keyboard in the open drawer, which, for me, is about the right height. This is so important because many people, believe it or not, work for hours, develop myofascial trigger points, and never think about the position of the keyboard or monitor. Keep your arms vertical or parallel with the floor. This is a good rule to follow. You may have to also adjust the height of the chair seat to accomplish this.

Also, if the chair seat is not the proper height, you'll develop trigger points in the muscles of your lower back and your legs. If there's too much pressure against the back of your legs for long periods of time, you could even develop phlebitis, or inflammation of the larger vessels in the legs.

Remember to get up and stretch every 20 to 30 minutes. Take a short walk. Drop your arms periodically and shake your hands to keep the circulation normal. Don't do what I do: keep going when you hurt, telling yourself that when you finish this page, you'll rest. Then continue to finish the entire document! Be smart and take care of yourself.

Table 13: Caffeine content of foods and medications

Product	Example	Caffeine Content (mg)
Chocolate	Baking chocolate (1 oz)	35
	Chocolate candy bar	25-30
	Cocoa beverage (6 oz)	10
	Chocolate milk (8 oz)	48
Coffee	Decaff (7 oz brewed)	3-4
	Decaff (7 oz instant)	2-3
	Drip (5 oz)	115-175
	Percolated (5 oz)	93-134
	Espresso (1.5 - 2 oz)	100
	Instant regular (7 oz)	65-100
Tea	1-Minute brew (7 oz)	40-60
	Instant (7 oz)	30
	Canned iced tea (12 oz)	22-36
	Iced (12 oz)	70
Soft Drinks (12 oz)	Jolt	100.0
	Sugar-Free Mr. Pibb	58.8
	Mountain Dew	54
	Mellow Yellow	52.8
	Tab	46.8
	Coca Cola	45.6
	Diet Coke	45.6
	Shasta Cherry Cola	44.4
	Shasta Diet Cola	44.4
	Mr. Pibb	40.8
	Dr. Pepper	39.6

Table 13: Caffeine content of foods and medications *(cont.)*

Product	Example	Caffeine Content (mg)
Soft Drinks (12 oz)	Pepsi Cola	38.4
	Diet Pepsi	36
	RC Cola	36
	Diet RC	36
	Diet Rite	36
	Canada Dry Cola	30
	Canada Dry Diet Cola	1.2
	Ginger Ale	0
	Hires Root Beer	0
	7 Up	0
	Barq's Cream Soda	0
	Big Red	0
Over-The-Counter-Drugs	Excedrin	130
	No-Doz Tablets	100-200
	Anacin	64
	Vanquish	64
	Midol	64
	Cold Relief Tablet	30
Prescription Drugs	Esgic	40
	Fiorinal	40
	Fioricet	40
	Darvon	32
	Norgesic	30
	Skelaxin	0
	Phrenilin	0

(References: (1) National Soft Drink Association; (2) Bunker and McWilliams. *J Am Diet* 1979;74:28-32; (3) Stavric et al.: Variability in caffeine consumption from coffee and tea: possible significance for epidemiological studies. In, *Foundations of Chemical Toxicology*, 1988;26(2):111-118.

Eight

Headaches

The most common complaint (perhaps next to hunger!), headache pain may be mild and short-lived, or its severity may totally incapacitate the sufferer. Fortunately, most headaches don't have a serious cause. In fact, chronic headaches are only rarely caused by such terrible disorders as tumors and aneurysms.

The term *headache* has been defined as the occurrence of pain or discomfort over the upper part of the head from the eyes to the back of the head. Actually, this definition is too restrictive; headache may originate in the face, teeth, neck, shoulders, back, or temporomandibular joints and then spread into the head as defined above.

Fortunately, headache pain in itself is usually not life-threatening. However, it's extremely frustrating to the patient, the patient's family, and the doctor. In one U.S. college town, 45% of those surveyed complained of headache ever week and 35-45% of them experienced headache severe enough to disrupt planned activities. Another survey conducted in a large U.S. city revealed that approximately 20% of women and 11% of men suffered severe headache pain. These statistics are similar throughout the world. Headache pain is a major problem for all of humankind.

In 1987, the National Headache Foundation estimated that more than ten million Americans suffered with some type of migraine and more than forty million with tension headaches.

As if headache pain wasn't enough, the economic impact is substantial. Headache sufferers account for more than 50 million doctor visits (medical doctors, dentists, chiropractors) per year, costing more than $400 million annually. When people suffer headaches at work, their efficiency is decreased. Next to back pain, headache pain accounts for more absenteeism than any other malady.

Migraine headaches rarely, if ever, last more than 24 to 36 hours. Many people who are diagnosed with migraine because their headaches are severe and last for days really don't have migraine headaches.

Although the International Headache Society divided all known headaches into 13 groups, there are three primary categories: vascular, traction/inflammatory, and muscle contraction. These are the divisions that we'll use in this chapter.

Vascular Headaches

Vascular headaches include, among others, migraine and cluster headaches. Because such headaches produce severe and frequently debilitating pain, all severe headache pain is often misdiagnosed as *migraine*. This is just not so. According to the International Headache Society, only 6-8% of headache pain is truly vascular. Yet, patients and doctors alike often term severe headaches — yes, you guessed it — migraine.

Most of the research money spent on headaches has been used to uncover the mechanisms that produce vascular headaches. It appears now that specific areas termed *receptors*, along with certain chemicals (neurotransmitters) are involved with migraine headache pain. Yet, with all the money spent each year on headache research, the only common trait known thus far is change in diameter of the blood vessels in the scalp and head. Also, certain foods and chemicals (for example, caffeine) are common to most migraine-type headaches.

Migraine headaches can basically be divided into two main categories: classic (migraine with aura) and common (migraine without aura). The major difference between these two types of headaches is the presence or absence of a time of warning (termed *prodromal phase* or *aura*) before the headache begins. If this aura occurs, the sufferer may experience visual symptoms (seeing stars, light sensitivity, water retention, periods of extreme creativity).

An intraoral splint is often effective in reducing the severity, duration, and frequency of vascular headaches. Splints also help reduce the muscle pain in the neck and shoulders after the migraine subsides.

Both the classic and common migraine usually begin before age 40 and often start in the teenaged years, especially for women. About six out of ten sufferers are women.

The migraine headache usually begins as a dull ache on one side of the head. As the pain intensifies, it builds in a crescendo fashion. Many people experience light sensitivity with migraine, which also intensifies, so that the sufferer would rather lie in a dark room, away from all noise and people.

The face may be pale or red and perspiring on the affected side. As time passes, the migraine headache intensifies from the dull ache to a pulsating type of pain. The pain may then spread from one side of the head to involve the entire head as well as the neck and shoulders. Nausea and vomiting are common. The pain is usually terminated by sleep.

This is a key point: **Migraine headaches rarely, if ever, last more than 24 to 36 hours**. As you can see, many people who are diagnosed with migraine because their headaches are severe and last for days really don't have migraine headaches.

Cluster headache. Another type of migraine headache is termed a *cluster headache* because the sufferers (usually men) experience headaches several times a day for several weeks, but then the attacks usually stop for a while. The episodes of attacks may even be seasonal; for example, pain only in the springtime or fall. Hence, the name *cluster* refers to a cluster of headache attacks. This type of headache has also been called a *histaminic* headache because the level of histamine in the blood appears to be elevated when the attacks occur.

A cluster headache starts suddenly, lasting from 30 minutes to 2 hours, and may wake the sufferer from a deep sleep. The pain is often accompanied by light sensitivity, tearing of the eyes and a running nose may be experienced.

Symptoms of cluster headache include pain on one side of the head, usually in or around the eye and the forehead and temple. The pain starts as a sudden attack, with little or no warning. The attacks, which last from 30 minutes to two hours, may even wake the sufferer from a deep sleep. The pain is often accompanied by light sensitivity, tearing of the eyes and a running nose. These headaches usually occur in men between the ages of 20 and 50 and often affect those who drink heavily or smoke.

Treatment for migraine (classic and common) and cluster headache is medication and dietary planning. Several foods are known to precipitate migraine headaches. If you suffer from this type of headache, you should avoid the foods listed in Table 14, as well as alcohol and smoking. If you do appear to suffer from vascular headaches, you should consult a neurologist.

One final note on vascular headaches: an intraoral splint is often effective in reducing the severity and frequency of these headaches. True migraine sufferers have a tremendous amount of muscle tension when the migraine occurs. If a splint is placed in the mouth, many report a decrease in frequency, severity and duration of their headaches. Also, splints help reduce the muscle pain in the neck and shoulders after the migraine headache subsides.

Table 14: Foods that may precipitate a vascular headache

Foods	Substitutions
Beer, red wine and sherry	No alcoholic drinks
Coffee, tea, soda with caffeine, hot chocolate	Decaffeinated coffee, herbal teas, caffeine-free soda
Smoked or processed meats (bologna, hot dogs, salami, sausage, pepperoni)	Freshly prepared meats
Chicken livers	Avoid
Pickeled herring	Avoid
Aged, tenderized or marinated meats	Avoid
Bananas, avocados	One-half per day
Papayas	Avoid
Broad beans and pods (lima beans, navy beans, pea pods, garbanzo beans, pinto beans)	Avoid
Citrus fruits (grapefruit, oranges)	One-half grapefruit, one-half cup of orange juice
Canned figs	Avoid
Nuts and seeds (sunflower seeds, sesame seeds, peanut butter, pumpkin seeds)	Avoid
Onions, sauerkraut	Avoid
Raisins	Avoid
Homemade fresh breads that are raised)	Avoid
Sourdough breads and crackers	Avoid
Chocolate	Avoid
Ripened cheeses (cheddar, Gruyere, Brie, Stilton)	American cheese, cottage cheese, ricotta cheese,cream and processed cheeses
Yogurt	One-half cup
Sour cream	Imitation sour cream
Fermented, marinated foods, MSG	Avoid
Buttermilk, chocolate milk	Avoid

Adapted from: Diamond S and Epstein MF. *Coping With Your Headaches* Chicago: Delair Publishing Co, 1982.

TRACTION-INFLAMMATORY HEADACHES

A second major category of headache pain is traction/inflammatory headaches. These are headaches produced by tumors, infections and inflammation inside the skull. The good news is that only about 2% of all headache pain is this type. The bad news is that this type of pain alerts the doctor that a serious and perhaps life-threatening problem may be present.

Sinusitis produces fever, nasal discharge, an increase in pain when bending over, and a general feeling of fatigue and illness. X-ray examination shows cloudiness in the visualized structure. This is never the case with vascular or tension headaches.

These types of headache are usually fairly constant, located in one place only and intensified by coughing, exertion, sudden head movement, bending over or even lying down. A patient with these type of symptoms, and in whom sinus or tooth infection has been ruled out, should see a neurologist.

Sinus headache. A rather common disorder, sinusitis, falls into this category of headache pain. Like migraine, *sinus* is often the diagnosis given a patient who is suffering from facial and headache pain. Frequently, doctors diagnose chronic, dull aching headache as *sinus*. It's very typical for a patient to tell me, "My doctor says I have sinus."

Unfortunately, this happens far too often, indicating that these patients have most likely been misdiagnosed and subsequently mistreated. Generally when someone mentions *sinus*, he or she means infection of the maxillary sinus. (The frontal, ethmoid and sphenoid sinuses may also be affected.)

All types of sinusitis produce fever, nasal discharge, an increase in pain when bending over, and a general feeling of fatigue and illness. In addition, an important test with any type of sinusitis is positive: x-rays. X-ray examination always reveals cloudiness in the visualized structure. This is never the case with vascular or tension headaches.

The type of sinusitis and its symptoms depends on the site of the infection (Table 15).

Table 15. Symptoms of sinusitis

1. Maxillary sinusitis causes pain and tenderness in the cheek area extending into the upper posterior.
2. With frontal sinusitis, the symptoms are forehead pain and tenderness.
3. An infection of the ethmoid sinuses produces pain in the eyes, swelling between the inner corner of the eye and nose and nasal congestion.
4. If the sphenoid sinus is infected, vertigo (a type of dizziness), coughing, eye pain, forgetfulness and mental dullness will be experienced.

As you can see, the symptoms of all these types of sinusitis hardly resemble migraine headache or TMJ pain.

Treatment of sinusitis includes the use of antibiotics, rest, pain medication, moist heat applied directly over the painful area and steam inhalations. If the infection persists, surgical treatment may be required.

Infections of the teeth. Teeth infections are also included in the general category of traction/inflammatory headache pain. Acute inflammation of the *pulp* (nerve and blood vessels) of a tooth produces toothache, especially when warm or cold temperatures contact the tooth. Frequently, headache pain will develop when an upper tooth is infected. This condition is often mistaken for maxillary sinusitis. The pain may be sharp, throbbing and shooting into the face, eye or head. Chewing, which produces contact against the infected tooth, will also produce severe pain. This problem is treated by removing the infection and repairing the tooth.

Headache can develop if an upper tooth is infected. This condition may be mistaken for maxillary sinusitis.

A chronic infection of a tooth will produce an abscess in the area of the root tip of the tooth. The abscess can spread into the bone and soft tissue, producing severe facial and head swelling, gnawing and continuous pain, and a temporal headache on the affected side.

Unlike acute tooth infection, the chronically infected tooth is soothed with cold liquids and ice. There are only two ways to treat this problem: extraction (removal) of the tooth or root canal therapy (removal of the dead pulp and replacement with a special type of root canal filling material).

Cranial nerve neuralgias. Neuralgias of cranial nerves are also contained within this general category of headache pain. As discussed in Chapter 6, trigeminal neuralgia is the most common type. However, *glossopharyngeal neuralgia* is another.

This neuralgia affects the glossopharyngeal (ninth) cranial nerve. Although quite rare in comparison to the trigeminal type, this neuralgia is very severe and debilitating. Symptoms include pain in the tonsillar area and ear that is of high intensity but of short duration. The pain is stimulated by swallowing, yawning, coughing, and tongue movement. A trigger area is often located on the side of the tongue.

Unfortunately, glossopharyngeal neuralgia may be confused with Eagles syndrome, a disorder of the stylohyoid ligament. Glossopharyngeal neuralgia can only be treated with neurosurgery.

TMJ headache. Headache due to TMJ is placed in the category of traction/inflammatory headache. This type of headache was discussed in Chapter 2.

Muscle Contraction Headaches

The most common type of headache is the muscle contraction or tension headache. This type of headache is estimated to account for 90 to 92% of all headache pain. Because tension headache pain ranges from mild to quite severe in intensity, it is sometimes misdiagnosed as migraine, sinusitis or even psychogenic (imagined) pain.

Because pain from tension headaches range from mild to quite severe in intensity, they are sometimes misdiagnosed as migraine, sinusitis or even psychogenic (imagined) pain.

Although classically the TMJ headache is placed in the category of traction/inflammatory headache, it most likely is of the tension type. Many reports in the scientific literature suggest that a displaced TMJ articular disc and temporal tendinitis both produce muscle contraction headache pain. Ernest syndrome may also produce this type of headache.

As a general rule, muscle contraction headache pain will depend on the emotional state of the patient. Psychosocial stressors contribute greatly to muscle contraction headaches. These stressors cause no direct physical injury like an injured TMJ or torn temporal tendon, but still, they are real causes of chronic, increased muscle tension with the subsequent development of neck pain and headache.

Stress is any physical or emotional factor that causes bodily or mental tension. Stress may be caused by job worries, financial problems, conflict within the family, death of a person close to you. However, stress can even be caused by positive changes in one's life: moving, achieving a personal goal, taking a vacation, a promotion at work. What psychologists have found is that stress is additive. The more stress in one's life, the more tension that person will experience.

Although stressful events vary from person to person, we can generally classify them into nine categories (Table 16).

Table 16. Common psychosocial stressors

1. **Conjugal.** Marital problems are often stressful, as we all know. Stress may result during the engagement period or wedding, from conflicts in marriage, separation from your spouse, divorce, or (probably the worst psychological stressor) death of your spouse.

2. **Parenting.** Did someone mention teenagers? Even the best kids present stressful problems, causing friction between them and you and between you and your spouse. Illnesses also certainly cause stress both concerning the specific situation and often between parents.

3. **Interpersonal relationships.** At times, stress develops even between the best of friends, associates, neighbors, in-laws, or employers. If these stressors are become chronic or unresolved, we experience muscle contraction of the neck and head muscles that produce muscle contraction headaches.

4. **Occupational stress.** Stresses today concerning down-sizing of companies, working longer hours, and more work being piled on everyone instead of filling a vacancy of a former fellow employee are common and affect most of us. Worry about the means to retire, or (if you're fortunate to be able to retire) simply adjusting to such a change in your life, are greater stressors than many of us really know.

Table 16. Common psychosocial stressors *(cont.)*

5. **Living circumstances.** Frequent moving, changing schools and churches, not to mention trying to find new friends, are very stressful and again, may produce chronic muscle contraction pain and frequent headaches.

6. **Finances.** As the cost of living continues to rise, or when inflation occurs, is it any wonder that so many of us have tension headaches? Living in debt and having no monetary reserves in the case of an emergency produce a muscle tension that underlies everything else for so many people today.

7. **Legal problems.** Pending lawsuits seem to never go away. The threat of financial loss, or worse yet, imprisonment certainly can cause muscle contraction headaches.

8. **Physical disorders.** Chronic illnesses, especially those that are undiagnosed (like TMJ) or concern for the need for surgery may cause a person to unconsciously tense their muscles, producing muscle contraction headaches that further add to the pain and stress of difficult situations.

9. **Injury.** Some of the worse cases of muscle contraction headaches I've seen in my practice are in folks who've been injured and are simply trying to cope with everyday life and still live as normally as possible. With problems that extend to finances, attorneys, insurance companies, doctors, employers, and families, it's no wonder that muscle contraction headaches result.

Because so many variables attribute to the development of muscle tension, symptoms may vary from one person to another. Nevertheless, muscle contraction pain usually occurs as a steady, non-pulsating ache. Vertigo, nausea, and tearing may also occur. Skeletal muscle trigger points may be present, usually in the muscles in the back of the head. The pain may involve one or both sides of the head and may occur at any time of the day.

Muscle contraction pain may last for hours, days, weeks or even months. Most people who have muscle contraction headaches realize that they are never really free from pain.

If headache is present upon waking in the morning, the probable cause is a muscle contraction headache produced by grinding or clenching of the teeth when sleeping. These type of headaches are frequently experienced at times of stress and high tension (hence, *tension* headache).

The pain of muscle contraction headache usually starts in the forehead, temples or back of the head and spreads over the neck and shoulders. Sleeping difficulties are common: waking without feeling rested, restlessness and trouble getting to sleep.

Those who clench or grind their teeth also develop muscle contraction headaches, especially during times of stress or during the night. When asking patients to describe their pain, I often hear such descriptions as tightness, drawing, band-like, or vise-like.

Muscle contraction pain may last for hours, days, weeks or even months. One patient I treated had suffered with a constant tension headache that varied in intensity for over 49 years. After proper treatment, her pain totally stopped within one week.

Most people who suffer with muscle contraction headache pain will realize that they are never really free from pain.

Another problem that often accompanies this type of headache is depression. This may be due to the nature of muscle contraction headache, but I really suspect the depression develops due to poor sleep, the constant pain like a dripping faucet, and the feeling that one is losing control of one's life with no relief from pain.

If headache is present upon waking in the morning, the probable cause is muscle contraction produced by grinding or clenching of the teeth when sleeping. Intraoral splint therapy is quite effective in these cases. Chiropractic therapy, dietary changes and reduction of stress are also helpful.

Treatment of muscle contraction pain should be aimed at the cause. For example, intraoral splint therapy is quite effective if a contributing factor is grinding or clenching of the teeth, which is often the case. Chiropractic therapy, dietary changes and reduction of stress are also helpful. At times certain muscle relaxants are required. Stress management with a psychologist may also be beneficial.

Often, just elimination of caffeine from the diet, changing posture at work, or relaxing will be more helpful than one could imagine. Exercise is also effective in reducing muscle tension.

One may need to use a combination of the above treatments. Also, realize that this type of headache is never really cured if it is a chronic problem. However, you can dramatically reduce the incidence and severity by following these suggestions.

Lastly, as with all pain problems, if you persistently suffer with headache and your doctor can't (or won't!) give you a reasonable answer, get a second or even third opinion.

Nine

The Concept of Pain

"Illness is the doctor to whom we pay most heed; to kindness, to knowledge we make promises only; pain we obey."

Marcel Proust

What Is Pain?

Before discussing the fascinating and complex topic of pain, we must define terms used by doctors and researchers who study pain. First, what is the definition of pain?

Certainly, hitting your thumb with a hammer causes pain; but what about toothache pain in a tooth with no nerve or leg pain years after its amputation? Also, are pain and suffering the same?

The concept of pain is fascinating; it has intrigued humankind since the beginning of recorded history. Pain commands humans to perform behavior that otherwise would be avoided. Pain may also be an ally of the sufferer — an excuse to avoid unpleasant tasks or situations when necessary. In addition, pain is a private experience: we can only measure the behavior of those in pain and not the pain itself.

Like pain, suffering is a private experience and yet it is a universally distressing sensation. Human beings and animals both have the ability to perceive pain. Animals can scream, howl, or run away from a painful stimulus. In humans, however, pain is far more complex. Each person may react differently to the same stimulus of pain. But why?

Researchers have tried to define pain for thousands of years, especially since the 1700s. A working definition of pain is "an unpleasant experience that we primarily associate with tissue damage." But tissue damage doesn't have to occur for one to experience pain. For example, phantom limb pain exists in an arm or leg that was amputated years earlier. So we might define pain as: "An unpleasant experience that we associate with tissue damage or *perceived* tissue damage."

Acute pain produces symptoms for our preservation; chronic pain is a disease in and of itself.

What are the differences between signs and symptoms of a disease? Like pain itself, symptoms are totally subjective. In other words, symptoms are what are reported by the sufferer. They can't be measured, only described. Signs, on the other hand, are objective: they can be measured by doctors or other health care personnel.

For example, you might say that you can't open your mouth wide because your right TMJ hurts. Limited opening is a symptom. How much do you mean? A doctor can measure the actual opening of your mouth with a ruler, thus observing a sign. X-ray findings and blood test results are examples of objective signs.

Although symptoms can't be measured, they are very important. They help paint a picture of different syndromes and diseases in the doctor's mind. Signs are important to help measure or gauge the severity of the disorder producing the symptoms. So when doctors refer to signs and symptoms, they mean what you say and what they observe or measure, respectively.

Acute pain

There are two general types of pain: acute and chronic. Acute pain is usually limited to the first few hours, days, or at most, up to six months after an injury. (Some researchers feel that acute pain can only last up to two weeks and then becomes chronic pain; however, this may be a little too soon for chronic pain to develop).

In addition to persistent pain, the chronic pain sufferer experiences a complex of psychological problems: sleeping difficulties, lack of energy, depression, decreased sex drive, anger, irritability, hostility and isolation.

Acute pain warns that injury has occurred, "announces" the location of the injury, and automatically directs the body to take protective actions. Examples of acute pain are burning your finger on a hot skillet, catching your finger in the car door, a broken tooth, fractured bone or a sprained ankle. Injury produces a series of physical and psychological events that are actually defense mechanisms for our preservation.

Have you ever twisted your ankle or broken a bone? If so, you noticed that your heart rate increased immediately, you may have become nauseated and even faint, or may have perspired a lot. If someone measured your blood pressure, it was elevated. The character of pain would have been sharp immediately, followed by a dull, deep aching. Swelling most likely would have occurred quickly after the injury.

In terms of your emotions, you may have noticed anxiety, anger or even feelings of loss of control of the situation. Your face probably showed classic expressions of pain: a furrowed brow, eyes squeezed shut, teeth clenched and a facial grimace.

Chronic pain

Like acute pain, chronic pain is frustrating, but usually more costly. Also like acute pain, the chronic type is associated with many physical and psychological side-effects. However, these are different than those of acute pain.

Although chronic pain has been defined as lasting longer than 6 months, many pain researchers now insist that chronic pain develops sooner than that. Whereas acute pain can be linked to a specific injury, the cause of chronic pain is often unknown. Acute pain can be termed a symptom; chronic pain is a disease in and of itself.

Chronic pain patients are often misdiagnosed as suffering from depression only. Although this may be one aspect of chronic pain, other factors must be addressed as well.

Depression in Chronic Pain

In addition to persistent pain, the chronic pain sufferer experiences a complex of psychological problems: sleeping difficulties, lack of energy, depression, decreased sexual drive, anger, irritability, hostility and isolation. He or she may have problems with weight gain or loss, depending upon the personality type. Further, the chronic pain sufferer may develop specific avoidance behaviors, especially concerning tasks and activities that he or she wishes to evade.

Unfortunately, these poor patients may become quite antisocial, angering family, friends and even employers. An additional problem with chronic pain is the potential for drug and alcohol use and addiction in an attempt to decrease pain and escape from its consequences.

The facial grimace of acute pain is absent; chronic pain patients exhibit depression and sadness on their faces. In fact, chronic pain patients are often misdiagnosed as suffering from depression only. Although this may be one aspect of chronic pain, other factors must be addressed as well.

Unfortunately, chronic pain sufferers often blame everyone, including doctors and therapists, for their altered life style and lingering pain. They frequently "doctor shop" and when disappointed, may employ an attorney to sue for malpractice.

Chronic pain also has its own language. It hurts. The pain is stabbing. It feels like a knife or an ice pick. There is pain and then intense pressure. At times, there's numbness and at other times, the pain is so sharp! All of these phrases could be used at various times to describe a TMJ problem, an injured back, or temporal tendonitis.

These are a few of the universal phrases that we human beings use to describe chronic pain. Scientific studies have shown that no matter what the language, when translated, all of us typically describe chronic pain with the same phrases.

Even though you might experience pain with normal activities, it is important to force yourself to engage in minimal activity, increasing the amount of activity each day. Walking and swimming in warm water are excellent activities.

Can you see why doctors have such a difficult time diagnosing the causes of chronic pain? They don't have a clue where to begin to investigate the patient's complaints. If your TMJ was dislocated in an accident and you had pain with a closed locked jaw, then you could point directly to the problem. The doctor would have no problem distinguishing the source of the problem.

However, it is different when pain has been present for months or years and the patient describes the pain as "like an ice pick in my ear" or "severe pain at times and then pressure like in an airplane." Where would you, as a doctor, begin to look for the problem? What seems so obvious to the chronic pain patient is obscure to the doctor and even worse, the patient's family and friends.

One recommendation often given by doctors, which actually contributes to the development of chronic pain, is bed-rest or inactivity for a long period of time. Even though you might experience pain with normal activities (such as chewing or talking with a TMJ problem), it is important to force yourself to engage in minimal activity, increasing the amount of activity each day. Walking and swimming in warm water are excellent activities.

Preventing acute pain from becoming chronic

Research is showing the importance of adequate treatment for acute pain. For example, studies of baby boys undergoing circumcision have found that untreated pain sensitizes the infant's central nervous system, which makes later painful experiences worse than they would be for other babies. In a comparison of infants who had been circumcised with those who hadn't, those who had undergone the procedure showed a stronger pain response to routine vaccination at 6 months.

Even though each of us is equipped with the same types of nerve cells, many other factors influence our concept of pain.

In another study, burn patients and their nurses recorded the severity of pain during painful procedures while in the hospital. Results showed that poor control of acute pain during these procedures correlated with significantly greater pain and poorer emotional adjustment after the patients were discharged from the hospital. The subsequent pain and emotional adjustment were not, however, related to total body surface that had been burned nor to the length of hospital stay.

Similar results were seen when patients undergoing surgery were evaluated. When patients receive pain medications before surgery, the severity and duration of pain is reduced in the postsurgical period. This regimen is called "preemptive analgesia."

One impediment to adequate pain treatment is the reluctance of patients to take medication for pain. In a 1997 report, 82% of over 1000 adults reported that they would not take drugs "fairly quickly" to stop pain. Many said that they would even wait until pain was "unbearable" before taking medication.

These studies highlight the importance of adequate treatment for acute pain. If you are in great pain or need to take large amounts of aspirin or Tylenol for more than several days, consult a doctor. Treat an acute TMJ problem with rest, a soft diet, ice (self-help measures described in Chapter 11) and suggestions your doctor may make. Do not perform the exercises in Chapter 11 until the acute pain and inflammation have resolved.

If a chronic pain problem develops, get a thorough medical evaluation from a doctor who is experienced in the treatment of pain. It is rarely "all in your head."

Do not allow, under any circumstances, any doctor to recommend surgery unless he or she can eliminate your pain with local anesthetic injections or demonstrate a pathological problem on an x-ray or MRI scan. Demand a second and even third opinion. It's your right, and if the doctor is sure of the diagnosis and recommended treatment, then no offense will be taken (or at least it shouldn't be!).

Culture plays an important part in the perception of pain and resultant behavior. In some cultures, it is socially acceptable to openly demonstrate suffering due to physical pain. In other cultures, one must exhibit a stoic attitude to even extreme injury.

Chronic pain sufferers are desperate and will do almost anything for promised pain relief. Do not fall into that trap! Make serious decisions about your treatment with a team of doctors and your family.

Remember: Every time surgery is performed, irreparable changes occur. Many are not good.

Pain Behavior

We've all heard of the soldier who, after being seriously wounded, still managed to perform an act of remarkable bravery without any concern for pain until after the danger passed. But then there's the person who appears to experience severe pain when sitting in the dental chair even though the doctor has done no more than touch a tooth. In contrast, some dental patients will allow any number of procedures without any use of local anesthetic and never flinch or blink an eye.

What is the difference between these people? As human beings, we all have the same types of nerve receptors that are capable of being stimulated. But why the wide range of diversity between the perception of pain between people?

Each of us has had different experiences; comes from different ethnic, social and religious backgrounds; and each of us has developed different attitudes about pain. These and other factors make the treatment of painful conditions very complicated.

We are indeed "fearfully and wonderfully made" (Psalm 139:14). Our nervous system is so complex that even the most complicated computer pales in comparison to the simplest cell in this remarkable system. Even though each of us is equipped with the same types of nerve cells, many other factors influence our concept of pain.

If you cut yourself when you were a year old and required stitches, chances are that anyone dressed as a doctor or nurse triggers a deep-seated fear or anxiety even today. As an adult you can usually be rational and control this fear when in the doctor's office but yet, the fear is still there. Why is your blood pressure elevated the first or second time the nurse takes this reading?

Can you see how an early experience of injury associated with terror can magnify a possible threatening or painful event later in life?

Many such psychological factors influence the way each of us handles a potential painful experience. Our relationship with the clinician is one. If you know and trust the doctor, nurse, or therapist, then chances are your reaction to a painful experience will be quite different than if you had no relationship with a new dentist or doctor in the emergency room.

Societal influences on pain behavior

What about the influence of your family? Perhaps in your family, pain was somehow optional. In other words, pain was "all in your head." Maybe your parents (because of their parents) taught you that to show pain demonstrated weakness, especially in public.

Another behavior of pain is total resignation to pain. In other words, people give up.

Our society as a whole rather admires this attitude. Think of action movies. The hero is often injured but rarely exhibits any pain behavior and continues to function almost as a "super-human." This and some parental attitudes can produce severe guilt in a person who genuinely has been injured.

Being one who has trained in karate, it used to be that I myself would never show pain in public even though my ribs were broken, not once, but twice! It wasn't the behavior of a karate master. That was how I was raised. "It can't hurt" or "real men don't cry."

As I grow older, I'm learning that real men do cry. However, due to my childhood experiences, this attitude has been a problem for me.

Also, it is no secret that "the bigger they are, the harder they fall." Those of us in pain management are bemused when huge, well-conditioned football players who give or take tremendous physical contacts in a game are terrified to visit the dentist. In contrast, I have seen small, frail women give birth without any anesthetic or sedative.

What's the difference? Certainly, the repair of a small tooth cavity can't compare (in a purely rational sense) to the obvious pain of a woman giving birth. Stature of a person has little to do with his or her perception of pain.

The large football player, normally under control of his body, has to totally surrender to the dentist for repair of the cavity, even though a local anesthetic has been given to assure that no painful stimulus will reach his brain. On the other hand, the small woman in labor, without any anesthetic to prevent painful stimuli from going to her brain, knows that pain is a part of giving birth, an expected and socially acceptable experience.

Depression is the component of chronic pain that is often termed suffering.

Further, with some people, "pain rarely occurs without an audience." In other words, some people exhibit painful behavior when around certain other people, but when they are alone seem to be fine. This is not always the case and this learned behavior is usually only a problem when taken to the extreme. However, there is "gain with pain" for some people; they perceive that their pain is far more unbearable than it physically should be. Whether actual or perceived (or both), the pain is real to the one afflicted.

Culture plays an important part in the perception of pain and resultant behavior. In some cultures, it is socially acceptable to openly demonstrate suffering due to physical pain. In other cultures, one must exhibit a stoic attitude to even extreme injury. Again, we all have the same anatomy for the perception of pain, but our cultures help mold us to the type of pain behavior that is acceptable.

In our culture, what happens when a child falls down and skins his knee? If a boy, usually he is told to "act like a man," "shake it off," and for heaven's sake, "stop crying!" But what if the child is a girl? Then we hold and embrace her, cuddle her closely and even encourage tears.

Can you see that these behaviors begin molding each of us from the beginning of life? My point is this: Each of us has had different experiences; comes from different ethnic, social and religious backgrounds; and each of us has developed different attitudes about pain.

Psychophysiology of Pain

These and other factors make the treatment of painful conditions very complicated. Because the temporomandibular joints part of the head, the center of our physical and emotional being, psychological factors like those described above have even a greater impact, generally, than the same magnitude of injury in the knee, for example. This is certainly true unless, of course, you make your living and derive your sense of accomplishment from playing professional baseball or football. Then, we can imagine, a knee injury of the same magnitude as a TMJ injury would be far more "painful" to the person injured. However, if you were a professional opera singer, then you would gladly accept a knee injury instead of one to the TMJ. Can you see how complicated the concept of pain is?

Depression often occurs partially as a result of undiagnosed pain. Many go from office to office and still suffer both physically and emotionally. Think what it does to them when they're told it's "all in their heads."

Another behavior of pain is total resignation to pain. In other words, people give up. They adopt a behavior of quitting their job, even if the pain is not debilitating. If offered part-time work, they will decline. They cease all hobbies or activities including visiting with family and friends. This person chooses to suffer in silence and ignores any sympathy offered by others. Actually, this type of behavior may well stem from attitudes of stoicism learned as a child. Solitude is deliberately chosen, imitating the loneliness of a child being punished by isolation.

This attitude of resigning to the pain is inevitable when continuing lack of relief only magnifies the pain, thus producing a state of constant suffering. This type of patient needs more than physical help.

Unfortunately, many who suffer with chronic pain develop another complex and frustrating illness:

depression. This is the component of chronic pain that is often termed suffering.

The term depression refers to a sad mood or emotion that may be a normal reaction to an important unhappy life event such as divorce or a business failure. With chronic pain, depression may be a normal development, distinctly different from the pain itself.

Doctors often prescribe medications such as amitriptyline, Desyrel, Paxil, Zoloft, Ambien, or Effexor for chronic pain patients to counteract increased neurotransmitters. Such medications may be just enough to improve a patient's sleep and outlook on life, which ultimately promotes emotional and physical healing.

Depression actually refers to a group of several psychiatric syndromes illustrated by long periods of constant, severe, and extensive mood changes. Initially, this depression is caused by an increase in production of some of the chemicals made in the brain (neurotransmitters). These chemicals produce personality changes and prevent the sufferer from obtaining a good night's sleep. In fact, the chronic pain patient develops an unconscious addiction to these, his very own neurotransmitters, and depends upon the personality changes which develop.

In addition to sleep disturbances, depression from chronic pain also affects work performance, sexual drive, and indeed, all other emotions. Depressed people feel worthless, tired, rise early in the morning, have slowed thinking, and may even have thoughts of suicide.

One final note on depression: it often occurs partially as a result of undiagnosed pain. As I have already mentioned, we conducted a study in which our office was the sixth, on average, consulted by patients for their pain complaints. These poor souls — and their families — had gone from office to office and still suffered both physically and emotionally. Most were told that the pain problems were "all in their heads." Have you ever heard that before?

This is especially true of those involved in motor vehicle accidents who are forced to file suit against insurance companies to have their medical bills and lost wages paid. They are accused of faking the pain and malingering. In fact, the doctors themselves don't believe these patients and frequently convince family members that there is no cause for such pain. Do you think these folks developed depression? Absolutely!

Some TMJ patients suffer from an anxiety disorder, in which their reaction to stress can disrupt and cripple their life. Anxiety disorders are illnesses. They frequently run in families but also may be related to the physiological characteristics and past experiences of the individual.

Doctors often prescribe medications such as amitriptyline, Desyrel, Paxil, Zoloft, Ambien, or Effexor for chronic pain patients to counteract the effects of the increased neurotransmitters. Such prescription medication may be just enough to improve a patient's sleep and outlook on life, which ultimately promotes emotional and physical healing. Certainly, referral to a psychologist, psychiatrist or social worker is advised for those severely affected with depression.

As I have stated, unless a pathological problem is found, no doctor can judge whether or not a person is experiencing tissue damage or perceived tissue damage. It doesn't matter: both produce pain with a resulting behavior. We can only observe the behavior and attempt to find the cause or causes of such behavior. However, it must be clear that pain is not a simple concept. It is influenced by learned behavior, social and ethnic backgrounds, and the influences of past experiences. All of this is in addition to possible or perceived tissue damage, not to mention the development of depression.

A person claiming to be in pain must be believed; we can only observe his or her behavior and not accurately measure his or her degree of pain.

I have observed that TMJ patients generally, but not always, experience their panic attacks while asleep.

Panic and Fear

Everyone knows what it's like to be anxious or really scared. Your heart pounds, the palms of your hands sweat, your pupils enlarge, and you either face the stressful situation or are able to withdraw from it. These reactions are normal and help us to react quickly to intense stress or fear.

However, some people, and frequently they're TMJ sufferers, also suffer from an anxiety disorder, in which their reaction to stress does just the opposite: it keeps the individuals from coping with the stress and can actually disrupt and cripple their life. Anxiety disorders are illnesses. They frequently run in families but also may be related to the physiological characteristics and past experiences of the individual.

There are many different types of anxiety disorders: obsessive-compulsive disorders, phobias, generalized anxiety, posttraumatic stress syndromes and panic disorder. The latter is the most common type that affects TMJ sufferers.

Those who suffer with panic disorder often wake at night with sudden terror. Without warning, they feel as if they're going to die; they may feel that their lungs have too much air in them; they may shake or tremble. Perhaps they feel as if they're choking or smothering.

The intensity and frequency of the attacks appear to be directly related to stress and to the severity of TMJ symptoms. Usually, the attacks only last a couple of minutes, but they can continue for as long as ten minutes or more. In rare cases, panic attacks may last as long as an hour.

When a panic attack strikes, the sufferers' heart begins to pound so intensely that they may think that it will burst. Their hands and feet might tingle or feel numb. They might even become dizzy and fall down. All sense of reality leaves and they know that, without a doubt, they're going to die. They might even think that they're having a heart attack or at the very least, losing their minds. Table 16 lists the common symptoms of panic attacks.

Panic attacks may occur at any time and any place. Some are plagued with these attacks while shopping or driving in traffic (termed agoraphobia). However, I have personally observed that TMJ patients generally, but not always, experience their attacks while asleep.

The National Institute of Mental Health states that at least 13% of the population suffer from an anxiety disorder, with about 12% of these being panic attacks. Women are affected about twice as much as men. These attacks may occur at any age, but usually they start in young adult life—late teens or early twenties.

Panic attacks frequently occur with those in chronic pain or those who suffer with depression, two terrible problems that plague many TMJ patients. To be diagnosed as suffering from panic attack, one must experience at least three attacks in a three week period.

The symptoms of panic attacks may also be precipitated by hyperventilation (rapid, shallow breathing). A person may become anxious for any number of reasons and begin to hyperventilate. As they do, the carbon dioxide level in their blood lowers, producing a temporary condition termed respiratory alkalosis. Symptoms of respiratory alkalosis are quite similar to panic attack: light-headedness, dizziness, numbness in the hands and feet, and feeling out of control.

At times, persons suffering with intense TMJ, facial and head pain may hyperventilate, thus producing panic attack-like symptoms. Also, drinking liquids with caffeine (coffee, tea, soft drinks) and some pain medications (see Table 13, page 90-91) that contain caffeine may also produce panic attack symptoms. So, just because you might have what appears to be a panic attack, it doesn't necessarily mean that you're going to be a life-long sufferer of this anxiety disorder.

Table 17: Symptoms of panic attacks

Symptoms of panic attacks
Intense, pounding heartbeat
Chest pains
Sweating
Terror
Fear of dying
Fear of falling
Shaking or trembling
Feeling out of control
Fear of going crazy
Flushing or chills
Shortness of breath
Feeling of being smothered or choking
Nausea or stomach problems
Lightheadedness or dizziness
Feelings of unreality

Adapted from: *Anxiety Disorders.* National Institute of Mental Health Publication No.94-3879, 1994.

If you think that you may be suffering from panic attacks, first consult your physician. Often, just knowing that you're physically healthy will be enough to ease your mind.

Many excellent medications can be prescribed for reducing or even eliminating these horrible episodes.

Further, you may ask your doctor to refer you to a psychotherapist for counseling, in an attempt to determine if there's another, often unrecognized problem, causing your attacks. Be assured that very often when your TMJ symptoms are reduced, your panic attacks, too, may reduce in frequency and intensity.

Those who are truly sane will seek help when necessary. It is not sane when individuals or their family members deny the problem exists and insist on "toughing it out" alone.

What can you do immediately if you experience a panic attack? First, try not to panic. Sit, or better yet, lie down. Try not to breathe too quickly (hyperventilation). Breathe into a paper bag. This will increase the carbon dioxide level in your blood by re-breathing your exhaled air. Yes, there's enough oxygen for you to breathe. Try to remember if you had consumed drinks, food, or medication that may have contained caffeine and if so, try to avoid these substances in the future. If the panic attacks continue, consult your doctor or a psychologist.

A Personal Confession

I understand a little about panic attacks because I'm a doctor who frequently sees patients with TMJ symptoms who report them to me. But my first introduction to panic attacks was a personal one: my wife is a sufferer of this terrible, torturous disorder, which usually visits her in the middle of the night.

When we were first married, I was an undergraduate student at Ohio State University. I was 20, my bride only 18, and she had never been away from home. Along with trying to cope with this new relationship, we also were awaiting my draft induction into the army during the Vietnam War. Needless to say, Cathy was stressed.

One night, about 2:00 a.m., Cathy suddenly awoke in terror, grasping her chest knowing that she was going to die. Her lungs felt too full — hyperventilation was very evident. "Help me! Help me!" she cried, with a look of fear on her face I'd never seen in the four years that we dated.

I'm thankful that our society is changing in its attitudes. Today most of us realize that emotional problems can be as crippling as physical diseases. With these attitude changes comes the revelation that no one should suffer needlessly from such disorders.

So what did I do, the "understanding, sympathetic, future doctor" who would dedicate his life to helping the hurting? I got angry, told her that she was crazy, and accused her of wanting to be with "Mother" more than me.

Plainly stated, I was a real jerk.

Obviously, my reaction to her dilemma didn't help and she continued to experience these attacks frequently. Cathy continued to suffer, and I continued my ignorant behavior. I finally made an appointment for us to visit a physician.

The doctor talked with us and immediately determined the correct diagnosis: panic disorder. She placed Cathy on medication, recommended some reading material, and counseled both of us.

The psychiatrist was right, and Cathy rapidly improved. My attitude, too, improved but it took many years, something for which I'm not proud. I didn't understand how someone who was so intelligent could act so irrationally, exclaiming aloud that she was going to die.

Well, perhaps you, too, or someone you know suffers from panic attacks. They're even worse when the attacks are coupled with TMJ problems. The attacks will pass, they will improve. There is hope.

I'm thankful that Cathy is so forgiving.

I'm also thankful that our society is changing in its attitudes. Today most of us realize that emotional problems can be as crippling as physical diseases. Most emotional problems can be treated, either with medications or psychotherapy or both. With these attitude changes comes the revelation that no one should suffer needlessly from such disorders and that those who are truly sane will seek help when necessary. The only real "weakness" or "irrationality" is when individuals or their family members deny the problem exists and insist on "toughing it out" alone.

How TMJ Pain Affects a Spouse

Also victims of TMJ are the sufferer's family members. Continuing a loving relationship with someone who has chronic pain is a constant challenge. As you can see in the following letter by the husband of a TMJ patient, everyone involved needs compassion and emotional support.

When treatment becomes difficult or the commitment to the recovery process overwhelming, patients should remember that they are not alone in their struggle.

I've tried to think back over the past 20 years that my wife suffered from TMJ pain and I began to remember things I wished would have remained forgotten. There is a very real "other side" to every story, and the TMJ spouse also has a story.

From a man's perspective, I think that one of the greatest problems is simply understanding the pain itself. Men for the most part perceive pain as having obvious visual characteristics. If you're not bleeding, bruised or limping, you must be fine. You get a headache, you take an aspirin and the pain usually goes away. You're as good as new, right?

When my wife would say, "You have no idea!" I'd think to myself, "Well, I've got news for you! I've known very severe pain before, too." I would actually take offense to a statement like that, like I didn't know what pain was. What I didn't realize was that my headache pain always went away after a while. Hers wouldn't. It may have subsided, but it never really went away.

It's no wonder she seemed distant, uncaring, indecisive, inattentive, and at times, downright hateful towards me. I took these attitudes personally for the longest time. The results were feelings of resentment, anger, distrust, regret, fear — you name it. But I also knew that this was not my wife and I also knew that this was not how she wanted to act and it certainly wasn't her fault.

There are so many spouses who "bail out" out of frustration. They don't understand what is happening to their spouse, and when combined with the normal day-to-day frustrations of family life, work, raising children, it's easy to see how life can become overwhelming to either spouse.

The good news is that I seem to be getting my wife back, and with that comes an unexpected "re-acquainting" process (both mental and physical). There were days when I felt that I was doing time for a crime I didn't commit, as though I had failed in some way. The problems really got deep and complicated, to say the least!

Brian Logan
January, 1996

Ten

Scleroderma

& Other Diseases that Affect the TMJ

Scleroderma is a rather rare connective tissue disease characterized by inflammation and excessive fibrosis (formation of fibrous connective tissue). This disease used to be known as "skin-bound" or "hide-bound" disease. Both terms describe the ultimate effects of thickening of the skin due to swelling and thickening of the underlying connective tissue due to an exaggerated production of collagen. (Collagen is the most abundant connective tissue fiber in the body.)

Scleroderma is not contagious and inherited only in rare occasions. The actual cause is unknown, but vascular, endocrine and autoimmune factors have been suspected.

About 19 persons per million are afflicted with scleroderma each year. Women are affected about three times more often than men, with an average age of onset of 40 years.

There are two types, localized and systemic (generalized). The localized form is usually not as severe as the generalized form.

Laboratory tests reveal an elevated serum levels of the enzymes glutamic oxalic transaminase, lactic dehydrogenase, and aldolase related to muscle involvement. Altered antibodies produce a positive latex fixation test in about 40% of scleroderma patients. In addition, there is an elevation in the erythrocyte sedimentation rate, and an increase in urine excretion of proline. These laboratory tests are positive for both localized and generalized scleroderma.

Localized Scleroderma

The localized type of scleroderma affects mainly the skin, but bones and muscles are also possible targets. Though not as severe as the generalized type, it does lead to a gradual decrease in joint mobility, the hands and TMJs being most affected. Also, calcifications form under the skin, and artery walls become rigid and thickened.

The localized type of scleroderma affects mainly the skin, but bones and muscles are also possible targets. Though not as severe as the generalized type, it does lead to a gradual decrease in joint mobility, the hands and TMJs being most affected.

Oral, facial and TMJ involvement

Oral manifestations of localized scleroderma include fibrosis of the tongue and soft palate, thinning of the lips and esophageal dysfunction. Neuralgia-like pain in the trigeminal nerve may develop.

When the facial muscles are involved, a progressive limitation of mouth-opening develops (microstomia) due to decreasing skin elasticity and narrowing of the lips. The nose may become pointed and seem to be covered with shiny skin (called "mouse facies"). The skin may draw tightly over the cheeks with the color appearing yellow-white or pale. The face becomes taut and hard as the disease progresses, resulting in a condition termed "mask-like" facies. Mobility of the eyelids and cheeks decreases.

The tongue may become smooth, along with development of a condition termed *frenulum sclerosis* (thickening of the attachment of the tongue to the floor of the mouth). This complicates routine cleaning of the mouth and teeth, and more frequent trips to the dental hygienist are needed.

When the TMJ is involved, pain, swelling and joint noise occur. Reduction of jaw movement may ultimately lead to the formation of adhesions and inflammation in the TMJs and destruction of the mandibular condyle and coronoid process.

TMJs affected by scleroderma destroy the normal occlusion (bite), which leads to the development of frontal occlusion (that is, biting primarily on the front teeth only). This change in the occlusion is caused by deformation of the surfaces of the mandibular condyle and articular eminence, the body of the mandible, and even the corner or angle of the mandible. Similar changes in occlusion are also common in such destructive diseases as rheumatoid arthritis and polyarthritis.

When the TMJ is involved, pain, swelling and joint noise occur. Reduction of jaw movement may ultimately lead to the formation of adhesions and inflammation in the TMJs and destruction of the mandibular condyle and coronoid process.

Biting on the front teeth causes severe tooth wear, sensitivity and even the death of teeth. But perhaps worse, such a forced jaw position worsens the TMJ symptoms, which make the occlusion worse, and so on.

Scleroderma is rare in children, but when they are afflicted, children seem to develop the localized form. It's fortunate that this localized form is not life threatening. However, significant facial deformity may develop, producing TMJ symptoms and problems, not to mention an orthodontic nightmare.

Systemic (Generalized) Scleroderma

Those affected with systemic scleroderma complain of being tired and depressed. Because they suffer with headaches, these patients are often seen in TMJ offices. Acrocyanosis (a circulation disorder in which the hands, and at times the feet, are persistently cold, blue and sweaty) is also a sign. This phenomenon, termed Raynaud's syndrome (bluing and cold feeling of extremities due to vascular spasms), develops in nearly all of those afflicted with this disease. It is often the first sign and symptom of scleroderma.

Be aware that Raynaud's syndrome does occur in about 3-5% of the general population, and does not necessarily indicate the presence of scleroderma.

Resorption of the mandible is more common than originally thought in those suffering with systemic scleroderma. Swiss researchers (Haers and Sailer) have reported that 20 to 33% of those with systemic involvement have mandibular resorption. Another 13% also have damage to the mandibular condyles. Women are affected sevens times more often than men. Such changes in the mandible certainly would affect the TMJs, the occlusion, and the muscles of the face, head and neck. No doubt, many of these patients also suffer with TMJ problems.

Doctors recognize two sub-types of systemic scleroderma: limited and diffuse.

Limited type of systemic scleroderma

The limited type is also termed the *CREST syndrome.* This acronym stands for the following combination of symptoms: **C**alcinosis (deposition of calcium), **R**aynaud's syndrome, **E**sophageal dysfunction, **S**clerodactyly (skin of fingers becomes stiff, smooth, and shiny), and **T**elangiectasia (dilated superficial capillaries) (Table 18).

CREST syndrome usually begins slowly, with the first symptoms appearing 10 to 20 years before all the symptoms manifest. The face, hands and fingers are usually affected first. The skin develops a diffuse, hard texture (*sclero* = hard; *derma* = skin), with the surface becoming smooth. Later, internal organs (e.g., the esophagus or lungs) become involved.

Table 18: CREST symptoms of limited scleroderma

CREST Syndrome	Symptoms
Calcinosis	Small, movable, non-tender, white calcium lumps under skin; NOT due to too much calcium in diet
Raynaud's phenomenon	Poor blood flow to fingers and toes due to spasms of the blood vessels
Esophageal dysfunction	Narrowing of the esophagus due to scarring of muscles; gastric reflux
Sclerodactyly	Skin of fingers and toes becomes hard and shiny; difficulty bending fingers and toes; contractures in fingers
Telangiectasia	Small blood vessels near skin surface become apparent, especially on fingers, palms, face, lips and tongue

Diffuse type of systemic scleroderma

Diffuse scleroderma occurs throughout the entire body. It often affects the skin and other organs. Depending upon the system involved, diffuse scleroderma may cause such disorders as hypertension, muscle weakness, kidney failure, bursitis of many joints (including the TMJ), gastrointestinal problems (bleeding, gastric reflux, and vessel damage), swallowing difficulties, shortness of breath, and difficulty grasping items or even typing. This diffuse type of scleroderma progresses at different rates in different people.

Many internal organs ultimately become involved with diffuse scleroderma (Table 19).

Table 19: Frequency of organ involvement in systemic scleroderma

Organ system	Percent involvement
GI Tract	90
Heart	50 to 90
Skin	90 to 95
Esophagus	50 to 80
Raynaud's Phenomenon	70 to 90
Kidneys	40 to 70
Lungs	40 to 90
Intestines	15 to 60
Joints	30 to 50
Anemia	30
Tendons	25
Skeletal Muscle	20
Hypertension	20
Pericardium	5 to 15
Stomach	10 to 30

Pregnancy

Pregnancy with systemic scleroderma may be uneventful. Both mom and the baby may do just fine. However, because scleroderma involves so many different body systems and complications do occur, careful prenatal planning is very important.

Women with diffuse scleroderma are at a greater risk for developing serious cardiopulmonary and kidney problems early in the disease. They should talk with their gynecologist and delay pregnancy if possible until the scleroderma stabilizes.

Fortunately, it doesn't appear that infertility or miscarriages are any more prevalent in women with scleroderma. Kidney problems seem to be the greatest risk, but unlike the development of high blood pressure in non-sclerodermic pregnancies, this problem has to be treated aggressively with scleroderma. In addition, sclerodermic pregnancies have higher percentages of intra-uterine growth retardation and premature delivery.

Women with diffuse scleroderma are at greater risk for developing serious cardiopulmonary and kidney problems early in the disease. They should try to delay pregnancy until the scleroderma stabilizes.

TREATMENT

Treatment of scleroderma is aimed at improving or at least maintaining joint range of motion and decreasing pain as much as possible. Physiotherapy under the guidance of an occupational or physical therapist is most helpful and effective. This includes movement exercises, medical massage therapy and underwater massages, swimming, walking, cycling, paraffin baths, chiropractic treatments, and the various types of myofascial release techniques. All these activities help keep the entire body flexible.

Exercise

Scleroderma patients should perform exercises to keep the joints and skin flexible. The following exercises should be practiced at least twice a day.

1. Follow the mouth-stretching exercise seen in Figures 17-19.
2. Slowly stretch your fingers on a table top, using firm and constant pressure.
3. Apply ice to the exercised areas when finished.

4. For specific exercises, consult a physical therapist, occupational therapist or a chiropractic physician trained in soft tissue therapies.

Protecting the joints

In addition to exercises, those with scleroderma should practice "joint protection" procedures. Protect painful and swollen joints — including the temporomandibular joint — from stresses and injuries with some of the following suggestions:

1. Avoid lifting heavy objects (I limit my patients to lifting no more than 10 pounds).

2. During times of painful and/or swollen TMJs, stick to soft foods (see Appendix C) and refrain from chewing gum.

3. Faithfully take the medicines recommended by your doctor, whether they are prescription or over-the-counter drugs.

4. Limit your activities; be sensible when performing physical tasks.

5. Consult the Arthritis Foundation's Guide to Independent Living for People with Arthritis for further information (see Appendix A).

Medications

Systemic treatment includes the use of antiinflammatory medications such as non-steroidal antiinflammatory drugs (aspirin, ibuprofen, Aleve, Naprosyn), glucocorticoids, and anti-fibrotic medications (penicillin infusions, gamma-interferon, and D-penicillamine). Antacids may be used to treat heartburn and to protect the lining of the esophagus. Also, medications for high blood pressure and drugs to reverse the decrease in blood flow of Raynaud's symptoms may be prescribed.

Amitriptyline (in low doses) may be useful in the treatment of peripheral neuropathy (nerve pain). Also, some researchers are experimenting with injecting skin lesions of scleroderma with interferon, which doesn't eliminate lesions but may stop new ones from developing.

Miscellaneous

Adhere to strict dietary changes. Eliminate caffeine and refined sugars, and maintain good oral hygiene. If oral manifestations occur, reduce foods with high carbohydrate concentrations. See your dentist on a regular basis to avoid developing periodontal (gum) and tooth problems, which otherwise can progress rapidly.

Protect your skin to maintain as good a blood supply as possible to your extremities. Dress warmly in cold weather. Wear a hat and cover your face and ears with a scarf. During winter months, use a humidifier to keep moisture in the air of your home. Avoid strong detergents and soaps that can irritate your skin and use moisturizing creams.

Try to manage your stress. Stress makes the symptoms of all chronic diseases, including scleroderma, far worse. Be sure to get enough sleep, which may mean taking short naps during the day. Consult a psychologist, social worker or counselor for assistance in stress management.

If you plan to have a baby, talk with your obstetrician first to protect both you and your baby. Obviously, it's best to become pregnant when your scleroderma symptoms stabilize.

For more information about scleroderma in general, contact the United Scleroderma Foundation (1-800-722-HOPE).

Giant Cell Arteritis (Temporal Arteritis)

Giant cell arteritis is an inflammatory disorder that affects the walls of large and medium size arteries, especially the temporal artery. Jaw weakness and pain when chewing or talking is experienced by 50 to 75% of patients with this condition. Other symptoms may include difficulty swallowing, aching in the temples or around the eyes, pain and stiffness throughout the body, loss of vision or double vision, scalp tenderness fever. Onset may be gradual or abrupt. Patients are almost always older than 60 years old.

Giant cell arteritis is diagnosed by a blood test called the erythrocyte sedimentation rate (sed rate) and by taking a biopsy of the temporal artery. This biopsy is a safe procedure performed under local anesthesia.

It is important that diagnosis and treatment of giant cell arteritis not be delayed. High doses of steroids will resolve the problem and prevent permanent and severe vision loss.

Tetanus

Tetanus is rare in the United States. However, those individuals who do not stay updated on their tetanus booster shots are at risk. One of the commonly presenting symptoms is trismus, a condition where the muscles of the jaw go into spasm, making it difficult to open the mouth. Trismus is also present in some temporomandibular disorders, so tetanus could be confused with a TMJ problem early in its course. It becomes difficult to swallow, and pain and stiffness extends to the neck muscles.

Tetanus can be cured if it is diagnosed early enough. The elderly and those who are immunocompromised (for example, individuals with leukemia or AIDS, or those taking immune modulators for cancer or arthritis) are most at risk.

Ehlers-Danlos Syndrome

A disease called Ehlers-Danlos syndrome is a connective tissue disorder that is characterized by joint hypermobility, and sometimes skin extensibility (stretchiness) and tissue fragility. These patients frequently experience chronic musculoskeletal pain that affects many joints, including the TMJ. Jaw hypermobility may lead to dislocation and degenerative changes in the condyle and damage to the discs. Many individuals with this disorder also suffer from chronic pain in their shoulders, elbows, hands, feet, knees and spine.

Cancer

TMJ pain may accompany many different kinds of cancer. Squamous cell carcinoma of the head and neck represent five percent of all cancers, and for men is the fourth most common type of cancer. It has been linked to heavy tobacco and/or alcohol use.

Sources of pain other than from the musculoskeletal system should always be considered when facial pain persists. Neoplasms in the head and neck regions may mimic TMD symptoms, or even be masked by a concurrent TMD. Sometimes a cancer that has metastasized from another site (for example, the lung) may exhibit its first symptoms in the TMJ.

If your pain persists or increases in spite of therapy, panoramic x-rays can rule out tumors in the mandible or maxilla. Luckily, tumors caught early can often be treated by radiation or surgery alone. Surgeries today are much less extensive, therefore less debilitating and causing much less cosmetic damage.

In a recent case report, a 27-year-old woman with a cancer called fibrosarcoma was misdiagnosed and treated for TMD for nine months before the cancer was diagnosed. Her symptoms included severe radiating pain, limited mouth opening, and numbness of the tongue and chin. Treatments during that nine-month period included occlusal adjustment, pain medications, trigger point injections, and physical therapy. When her symptoms worsened, a CT scan of the left neck revealed a large soft tissue mass. She underwent wide excisional surgery, chemotherapy and radiation therapy.

Luckily, there are specific signs and symptoms to look for to differentiate TMJ disorders from cancer. If you notice any of the following, be sure to bring them to the attention of your doctor and/or dentist.

Table 20: Symptoms of head or neck cancer

1. Neurologic signs, such as numbness
2. Auditory complaints
3. Constant pain unrelated to jaw movements
4. Unchanging or worsening symptoms in spite of several different treatments
5. Lymphadenopathy (swelling of the lymph nodes in the neck or armpits)
6. Symptoms such as nosebleed, nasal stuffiness or drainage, or difficulty swallowing
7. Rapid onset of trismus (muscle spasms in the jaw that make it difficult to open or close the mouth)
8. Unexplained weight loss
9. A mass or lump in the orofacial or neck region

Individuals who have undergone bone marrow transplantation or total-body irradiation to treat childhood cancers may have a high prevalence of TMJ symptoms as adults. Movement and function of the TMJ may be limited, and the masticatory muscles may be tender. Mouth opening may be limited.

Ankylosing Spondylitis

Ankylosing spondylitis is an inflammatory arthritis that affects the spine and nearby structures. The TMJ is affected in about half of these patients. The jaw may be hypermobile, and bone deformation may be seen in the condyle.

Bursitis of the Pterygoid Hamulus

This condition may present with pain in the ear, throat, and upper jaw. It is caused by trauma, such as swallowing a large bolus of food or wearing a denture that is too long in the back. Treatment with steroids and NSAIDs may resolve the problem, but surgery may be required if conservative treatment doesn't work

Meniere's Disease

This is a disease of the inner ear. Symptoms include periods of dizziness, ringing in the ear (tinnitus), and occasionally deafness. The *Journal of Orofacial Pain* has reported that patients with Meniere's disease are more likely to have pain in the face or jaw and impaired TMJ function.

McArdle's Disease

McArdle's disease is one of the glycogen storage disorders that affects skeletal muscle. It is characterized by muscle pain, weakness, and tenderness. These patients will suffer muscle cramping during exercise, but may experience "second wind" phenomenon, in which they may return to exercise after a brief rest with no tissue soreness. This is because their body cannot produce lactic acid in the muscle tissues, which normally makes our muscles sore after exercising.

The condition is usually diagnosed during late teens. Patients with McArdle's disease may experience pain of the TMJ, muscle tenderness, and restricted jaw opening.

Cysts

Pain in the area in front of the ear may herald the presence of a cyst or mass within the TMJ. These benign growths may include ganglion cysts, synovial cysts, and osteochondral loose bodies. Loose bodies are comprised of bone and cartilage.

Symptoms may include swelling and pain in front of the ear, hearing loss, TMJ pain, and/or decreased mouth opening. It may be difficult to close the teeth together, and the mouth may deviate to one side when opening or closing. Treatment is usually surgery, and outcome is almost always excellent.

Juvenile rheumatoid arthritis (JRA)

JRA is a chronic synovial inflammation in children that can cause facial and TMJ deformities. About a third of these patients will have a "birdlike" facial appearance (called micrognathia). Unfortunately, damage can occur before clinical symptoms begin. Therefore, children with JRA should be examined regularly by their dentist.

Lupus Erythematosus (LE)

Lupus erythematosus is a connective tissue disease that has the potential to affect many organ systems. Symptoms include rashes, oral sores, kidney disease, anemia, arthritis, and increased risk of heart disease. More than 75 percent of these patients have oral problems, such as dry mouth, burning mouth, oral ulcers, and periodontitis. Symptoms may resolve for periods of time and then recur. Treatment includes steroids and immunosuppressant drugs.

Up to 60 percent of patients with systemic LE have TMJ problems. A flat-plane occlusal orthotic may be recommended to "unload" the joint and to prevent further joint injury.

Lyme Disease

Lyme disease is transmitted by ticks and affects the skin, nervous system, heart, skin, and joints. Symptoms include chills, fever, headache and joint swelling. Antibiotic therapy is usually advised. If the jaw is severely affected, trigger point injections into the aching muscle may help.

Parkinson's Disease

Patients with Parkinson's disease may have impaired orofacial motor control and muscle rigidity. This may lead to orofacial pain and muscle fatigue, TMJ discomfort, cracked teeth, displaced tooth restorations, and tooth loss.

Physical therapy and a splint worn at night and during times of increased stress will help with these symptoms.

Infection

A simple measure to rule out infection as a cause of TMD symptoms is to take your temperature and to feel for swelling in the lymph nodes of the neck. Infection may be accompanied by chills, trismus, swelling at the angle of the jaw, and bulging in the throat.

Septic arthritis is a bacterial infection and resulting inflammation of the jaw joint. Sometimes the infection will begin elsewhere in the body and spread to the TMJ. Symptoms include stiffness, tenderness, pain, warmth and swelling.

Usually antibiotics are required to clear an infection. In recalcitrant cases, incision and drainage of the abscess or surgery may be required.

Eleven

Self-Help

As with any joint or soft tissue injury, patients can perform self-help measures at home. In patients suffering from a TMJ problem that requires treatment, self-help procedures probably won't cure but certainly can reduce pain.

For any number of reasons, people choose not to have TMJ treatment: expense, inconvenience, inability to find a TMJ specialist or other commitments. The pain and dysfunction may not be bad enough to require treatment. In many cases I first suggest that the patient follow some home treatment techniques mentioned in this chapter before they commit to treatment.

Even if you undergo successful TMJ treatment, there will be times in your life when you won't be able to see the doctor for treatment — and you shouldn't every time you hurt. At those times, self-help tips are important in reducing your pain as quickly as possible yourself. Just as Jim Downard (see Foreword) has learned to use self-help measures when he has minor recurrence of pain, you too will want to know how to minimize your pain should it return.

Rest

Physical pain tells us that we probably have been injured. Pain in the TMJs tells us that we must rest the joints and give the body time to heal. If you have a splint, place the splint in your mouth to separate your teeth. Relax your facial muscles, and if you clench your teeth, make a conscious effort to stop.

Those in a church choir or a singing group should take a leave of absence and allow the joints to heal. Just as well-conditioned athletes must at times refrain from play, if you don't give your body a chance to heal, a more severe problem may develop.

By the way, if you play a reed instrument or scuba dive, don't. Both activities put a lot of strain on the muscles that control the TMJs and can make the pain worse.

I often suggest that patients follow some self-help techniques before they commit to treatment. Even if you undergo successful TMJ treatment, there will be times in your life when you won't be able to see the doctor — and you shouldn't every time you hurt. At those times, you will want to know how to minimize your pain.

Soft Diet

When you're having TMJ pain, even if you're undergoing active splint therapy, you must adhere to a soft diet. The temporomandibular joints are capable of withstanding heavy forces during chewing, when they are healthy. But when inflammation or injury to the joints occurs, you must reduce the forces generated during chewing. Even if your problem is not in the joint per se, tough or fibrous foods put a tremendous amount of strain on the muscles, ligaments and tendons.

Avoid hard and tough foods like raw carrots, apples, tough meats, salads and nuts. Refrain from bakery goods like bagels and dinner rolls. Use a blender to grind tougher foods so that your nutritional requirements will be met. See Appendix C.

Limiting your Opening

When a joint hurts, a protective mechanism called *muscle splinting* automatically occurs. This neurologic reflex is for our benefit: an acutely injured joint hurts and shouldn't be moved through its full motion. Likewise, when your TMJs hurt, they too should not be moved any more than necessary. The muscles that open and close the joints will be sore and even painful. You must limit jaw movements to rest the joints and to avoid producing more muscle and joint pain.

Therefore, don't force your mouth wide open. Avoid eating large sandwiches, whole apples, whole peaches or any other food that requires a wide opening of the mouth.

If you play a reed instrument or scuba dive, don't. Both activities put a lot of strain on the muscles that control the TMJs and can make the pain worse.

Avoid Prolonged Opening

It is also important to avoid having your mouth open for a long period of time. Normally, you don't. But, have you ever had your teeth cleaned or had a crown placed on a tooth? Then you know how long you have to keep your mouth open.

For some people, the stress of going to the dentist can make their jaw muscles tense even before they open their mouth. Then, if the doctor or hygienist has to perform a long procedure, their mouth will be open and pressure will be placed against their lower jaw. These can all contribute to a TMJ problem, especially if you're already suffering with one.

Explain to your dentist or hygienist that you have a TMJ problem and ask to rest your mouth every few minutes. Avoid any unnecessary procedures such as placing a crown for esthetic reasons only. Also, avoid having your wisdom teeth removed unless absolutely necessary. Even the easiest extractions produce tremendous pressures on the joints and jaws. Your dentist may offer to place a bite block between your teeth to minimize the stress. This device will reduce the stresses on your muscles and joints.

Start taking aspirin (600-1000 milligrams) every 6 hours or ibuprofen (600 milligrams) every 6 hours the day before your appointment, the day of your appointment, and the day after your appointment. This will reduce swelling, pain and inflammation in the joints.

Your mouth will be open with a lot of pressure against your jaw during a long dental procedure. Take aspirin or ibuprofen every 6 hours the day before your appointment, the day of your appointment, and the day after.

If you are allergic to aspirin or ibuprofen or if you have stomach problems, then take 1000 milligrams of acetaminophen every six hours the day of your appointment (no need to take acetaminophen the day before because it has no effect on the process of inflammation) and every six hours the next day. Although it won't stop inflammation, this drug will reduce your pain.

As soon as possible after your dental appointment, apply icebags over both TMJs (25 minutes on and 5 minutes off) for a few hours after the appointment. Then use moist heat several times that evening and the next day (if necessary). By following these simple steps, you'll greatly minimize any flare-ups of your TMJ problem.

Ice or Heat?

One question I hear a lot is, "When my joints hurt, do I use ice or heat?" The answer is "both."

As with any joint injury, apply ice immediately after an injury to reduce swelling and pain. Continue to use ice for at least the first 12 to 24 hours. An ice bag can easily be made from a zip style plastic bag. Place the ice bag in a wash cloth or dish towel and then place the cloth over the TMJ. Apply ice for 20 to 25 minutes and then remove for about 5 to 10 minutes. Repeat this for several hours.

Heat, on the other hand, is quite effective after the first 24 hours following an injury. Moist heat, due to its deeper penetration, is more effective than dry heat. Purchase moist heating packs at a drug store. You can also make a moist heating pad from a dish towel. Soak the towel with water and wring dry. Then place the towel in a microwave oven for 30 to 40 seconds — be careful not to burn yourself. When tolerable, place the heated towel directly over the painful area until the heat dissipates. Repeat this procedure as often as possible. (But don't burn your skin!)

As with any joint injury, apply ice immediately and use for at least 12 to 24 hours to reduce swelling and pain. Heat is quite effective after the first 24 hours following an injury.

Many patients are touting their homemade "rice socks." To make one yourself, place about two pounds of uncooked, regular (not instant) rice into a clean, 100% cotton tube sock and knot the open end. (Avoid those socks that could use some darning!) Microwave your rice sock on high for about 3 minutes. (Some trial and error will be necessary here to get it just the right temperature: kind of like popping popcorn to get most of the kernels popped without burning it!) You then drape the sock under your neck and over both TMJs. This heat pack will retain heat for about half an hour, and it can be reused over and over again. People with arthritis and fibromyalgia may find many muscles and joints that will benefit from rice sock therapy!

A long-lasting moist heating pad can be made from an electric heating pad, a plastic bag, and a moist towel. Wrap the electric heating pad in the plastic bag. Moisten a towel and wring it out. Place the towel around the plastic bag (which is around the heating pad) and turn the control on medium. This will provide penetrating moist heat for a long time.

One word of caution: Don't fall asleep with the heating pad on. You could burn your skin or have an electrical problem.

If you're experiencing swelling, use ice and not heat. Ice is best to reduce to stop swelling and pain.

Good Nutrition

Healing demands good nutrition. For example, when connective tissue is injured in a joint or ligament injury, the protein collagen, which is the main framework of connective tissue, must be repaired. Vitamin C is necessary in the production of collagen and therefore, during times of injury, the body's demand for this water soluble vitamin increases. Other minerals such as calcium, magnesium and zinc are necessary for proper muscle activity and health. Also, the complex of B vitamins supplies many needs in normal body metabolism and especially during times of stress, both physical and emotional.

More information about nutrition is in Chapter 13.

Posture

Good posture is important for many reasons, especially to the TMJ patient. Scientific studies have shown that posture affects head position, and head position affects mandibular position. As you can imagine, the position of the lower jaw has a great influence on the discs in both joints. For muscles in the head, neck and back to be in balance as they were created, you must strive to maintain good posture.

Shoulder height. Have you ever developed a back or neck ache while sitting at a computer or typewriter for a long time? Did you also notice that simply by changing the position of the monitor or keyboard, your pain stopped? Just imagine if your posture was poor continually. One thing you can do to help reduce TMJ pain is strive to improve your posture.

Women who carry diaper bags or large purses on their shoulder develop shoulder, neck and head pain simply due to a self-imposed poor posture. Carry these bags in your hand and not on your shoulder (Fig. 14).

When carrying bags of groceries, for example, keep them light — no more than 5 - 7 pounds — and close

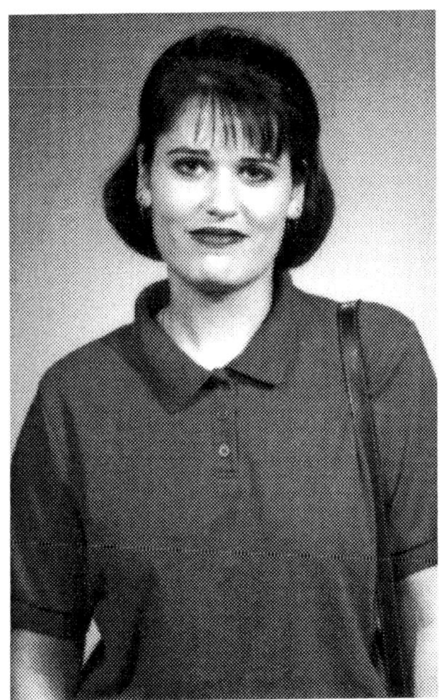

Figure 14: Elevation of shoulder that aggravates TMJ symptoms

to your body, not out in front. Also, don't reach far forward for an object or bend over to pick an object up. Move in closer or squat down before picking something up, including the kids!

Sitting posture. Avoid sitting too close to a speaker or a movie screen. Tilting your head back will cause your neck muscles to overwork, thus causing pain in the head and neck.

Also, understand that chairs are not really designed for our comfort. They supply little or no middle back support and this produces an unconscious forward head and shoulder posture. You can help yourself at work by placing a small pillow between the small of your back and the chair.

Poor back support also occurs when driving or riding in a car. If the seat is tilted back too far, you'll develop neck and head pain from leaning forward.

Place a small pillow or cushion between your back and the car seat. If the seat is tilting too far forward, then neck pain will develop from trying to hold your head up to keep your eyes on the horizon. Lean the seat back to a more comfortable position. Keep your entire back supported when sitting.

Standing posture. Most of the postural muscles of the body are related to each other in some fashion and all are related to the mandible and its muscles. Strong leg muscles attach to the bones of the legs and pelvis; lower back muscles attach to the pelvis, spinal vertebrae and ribs; upper back muscles attach to vertebrae, ribs and the shoulder girdle; these muscles, in turn, attach to the base and back of the skull.

If any of these muscles are injured or not working properly, the head's position is affected, which in turn affects the jaw position. Therefore, it's very important to maintain correct standing posture.

For human beings to stand erect, the muscles in back of the body have to work in coordination with those in the front. Part of those front muscles are the muscles of mastication (the muscles that open and close the jaw). These muscles help hold the head over the shoulders. If in pain or dysfunction as frequently happens with TMJ, the jaw muscles must overwork, thereby producing even more muscle pain. Even worse is that the overworking of the jaw muscles can actually cause jaw displacement and further TMJ damage.

If you stand for any length of time, put one foot up on a stool or step. This will reduce the development of pain in your lower back.

As with sitting, avoid placing your head forward of your body when standing. This produces an increase in muscle activity of the back and neck muscles. Your head weighs about 12 pounds (lighter for some of us!).

Concentrate on your head position. Try to keep your head erect, placed directly over your shoulders

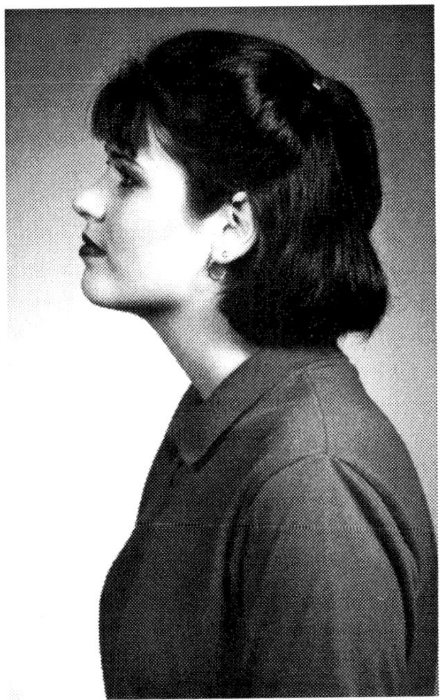

Figure 15: Forward head posture

and not in front of your body. If your head hangs in front of the body (Fig. 15), then the jaw closing muscles and the neck muscles will have to over-work, which produces pain and referred pain.

This does not mean that you should stand "at attention" or pull your shoulders far back. This posture, too, can produce muscle pain. Relax your shoulders and chest so that your head is balanced without pull or strain of any neck muscles.

Just imagine walking around with a 12-pound weight held in front of your body. It would not be long before your lower back and neck would react, the muscles would probably go into spasms, and the head and jaw positions would be unnatural and therefore, not healthy. Trigger points would develop and before long, your entire back, neck and even legs would be painful, just because of the weight held in front of your center of gravity.

For the TMJ patient, this postural problem is even worse. In this example, the head would be thrust forward. We're created to keep our eyes on the horizon and therefore, with the head position forward, you would have to tilt the head back as well. This would produce even more muscle fatigue and pain in the shoulders and neck and more important, the lower jaw would be forced backwards in the TMJs. This could produce inflammation, swelling, pain and even discal dislocation in one or both joints. The resulting change in occlusion would produce tooth sensitivity and bruxism.

Can you see how this could make the TMJ problem worse? Therefore, it is very important that all of us but especially you, the TMJ sufferer, keep your head erect over your body and avoid any type of forward head posture. Physical therapists and chiropractors are excellent to consult for this problem.

Avoid lifting any object weighing more than 3 to 5 pounds (including your children, mothers!) without first squatting down and lifting with your legs.

Phone use. Another postural problem occurs when we hold the phone between our jaw and shoulder, trying to take notes or a phone number. If you engage in this activity for any length of time and certainly if you have a TMJ problem, then you must stop holding the phone this way.

Just like forward head posture, tilting the head to one side to hold a phone develops trigger points in the upper back and neck muscles (Fig. 16). These trigger points will produce pain and limitation of neck and head movements which ultimately may alter the jaw position, injuring the TMJs. This is a frequent problem for receptionists. Buy a headset — they are very inexpensive — and you'll solve this problem.

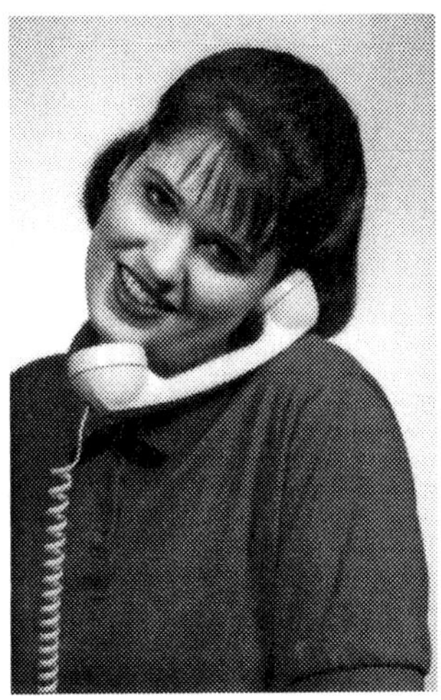

Figure 16: Improper way to hold phone

Jaw Exercises

One word of caution: You should check with your TMJ doctor prior to doing any of these exercises. He or she may not want certain exercises performed at this point in your treatment.

These exercises help reduce muscle and joint pain. They should be done slowly, without a jerking or quick motion. Also, apply moist heat over your TMJs and jaw muscles for a couple of minutes before attempting these exercises. When finished, apply ice over the joints and muscles for about ten minutes.

1. Opening and closing. One easy yet effective exercise is performed by placing half a toothpick between the upper two front teeth and the other half between the lower front teeth. Looking in a wall mirror, slowly open and close, concentrating on keeping the toothpicks in a straight line (Figure 17). Repeat this exercise 20 to 25 times, 3 times per day.

2. Opening against resistance. Sit at a table, place your fist under your chin, and rest the weight of your head on your fist. Open your mouth slowly five times, rest, and repeat (Figure 18). Repeat three times a day.

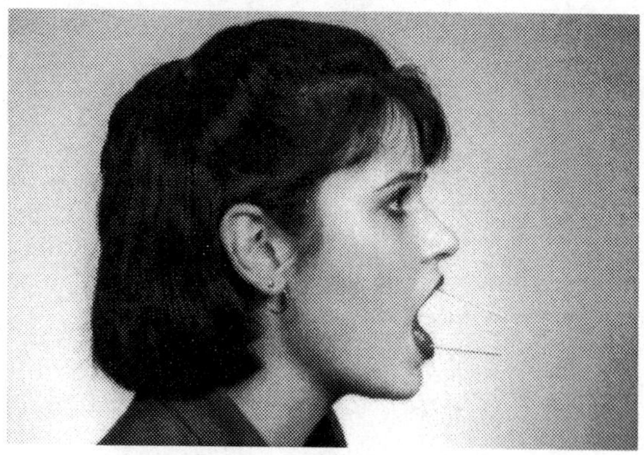

Figure 17: Opening and closing

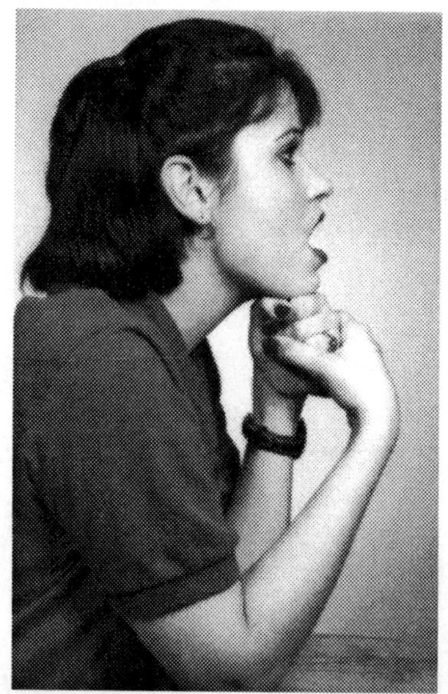

Figure 18: Opening against resistance

3. Opening and closing against light resistance. To strengthen both opening and closing muscles of the jaw, apply light pressure against the chin with opening and closing. Using your thumb, lightly push backwards against your chin as you open and close (Figure 19). Repeat ten times, rest, and repeat again. Don't use strong pressure. The goal of this exercise is to

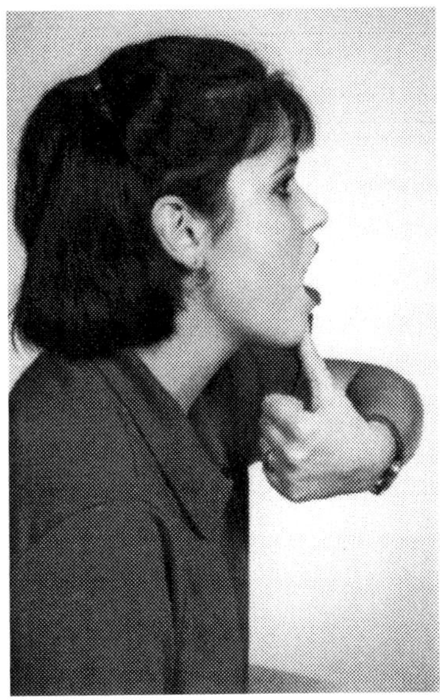

Figure 19: Opening and closing against light resistance

open and close against light, not heavy resistance. Pushing too hard could produce joint pain and even swelling.

Neck Exercises

Because the neck muscles position the head and have so much effect on the TMJs, it's important to exercise and strengthen them as well. All of the following neck exercises should be performed in front of a mirror either sitting in a chair or standing erectly.

If possible, it's good to do these exercises while standing in a hot shower. The moist heat will improve blood circulation in the postural muscles, thus making the exercise sessions more effective.

1. **Side bending of the head.** This exercise stretches the neck and upper back and helps to improve posture. With your arms to your side, gently tilt your head to one side as if you were going to touch your ear to your shoulder. Inhale while doing this.

Then, while exhaling, slowly bend your head further, attempting to bring your ear as close as possible to your shoulder without causing opposite neck pain (Figure 20). Hold that position for five seconds. Repeat this exercise to the other side. Repeat five times to each side, three times per day.

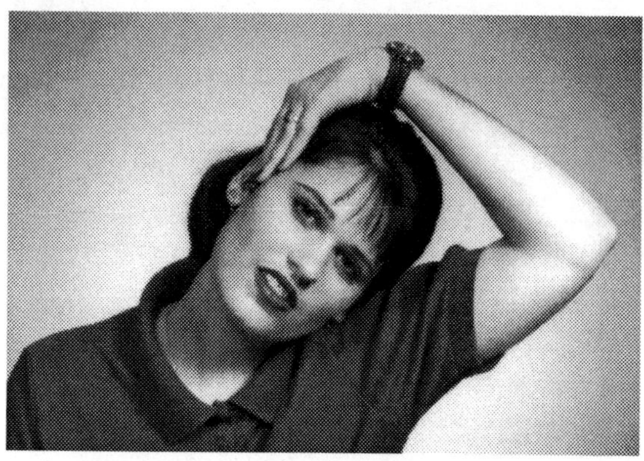

Figure 20: Side bending of the head

2. Head rotation. This exercise stretches many of the neck muscles and improves the range of motion of your head. With your hands at your side, slowly exhale and turn your head to one side as if you're going to look over your shoulder. Turn as far as possible and hold this position for five seconds (Figure 21). Repeat this exercise to the other side. Repeat five times to each side, three times per day.

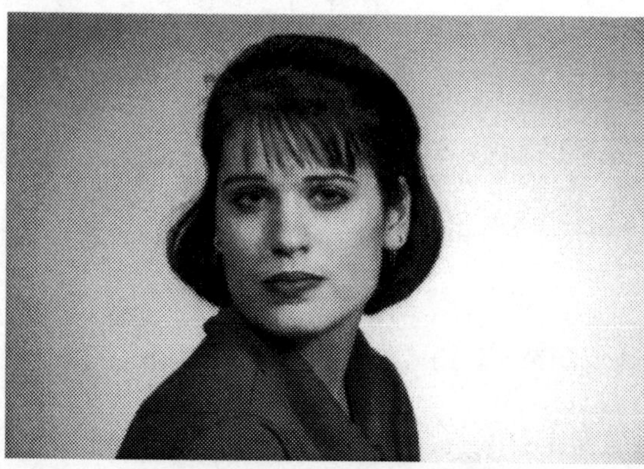

Figure 21: Head rotation

3. Head flexion. This is a good exercise to stretch the upper back and neck muscles, which decreases neck and back pain and improves posture. Inhale. Place your hands on the top of your head. Exhale slowly and gently drop your head as if your were going to touch your chin to your chest (Figure 22). Keep your mouth closed. Gently pull downward with your hands to increase the stretching. Hold this position for five seconds and slowly return your head to its normal position. Repeat five times, three times per day.

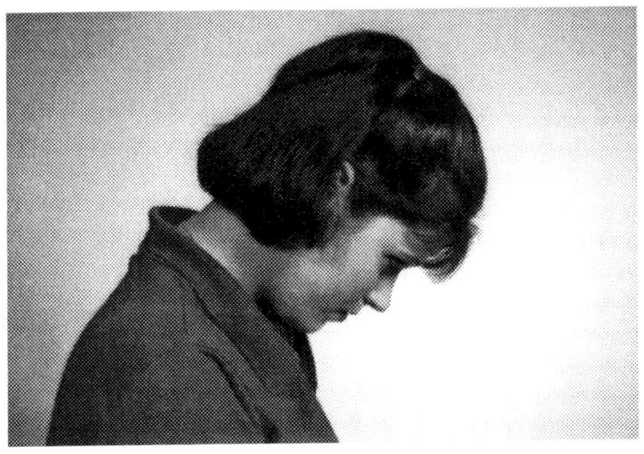

Figure 22: Head flexion

4. Shoulder stretching. For this exercise, you must stand up. If you're going to do this exercise in the shower (the hot water is very therapeutic), then you grasp either the shower head or the top of the shower door with one hand. If not in the shower, grasp the top of a door (Figure 23). Inhale and gently "hang" on your arm (keep your feet on the floor!). While hanging, slowly exhale and then hold that position for five seconds. Repeat with the other arm. Do each of these five times, three times a day.

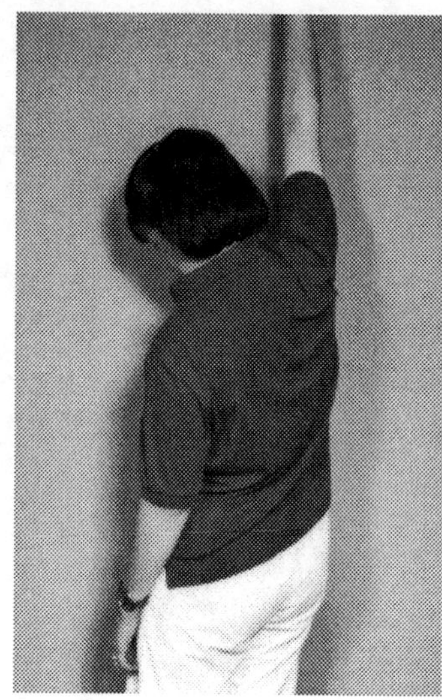

Figure 23: Shoulder stretching

General Exercise

General exercise is good for everyone, but especially those suffering from TMJ or other chronic pain problems. This type of exercise is meant to mobilize the entire body, not just an isolated area like the jaws.

Physiologists tell us that exercise releases chemicals from our brains (natural pain killers called endorphins) into our blood. Psychologists report that exercise helps us deal with stress and combat depression. Plus we all know the physical benefits of exercise. Think of it this way: when you exercise, you get three times the "bang" for your buck !

If you suffer any type of chronic pain, you can't afford to become sedentary; you'll gain weight, become depressed, and simply lose hope. You must commit yourself to some type of exercise, no matter how non-physical it may seem. Start slowly, and gradually build your endurance.

Walking is one of the best and simplest exercises you can do and can even be done inside a shopping mall during bad weather. Again, the goal is not to walk a "5 minute mile;" no. Start slowly, attempting to walk about one mile in 20 to 30 minutes three times per week. When you can, increase your speed so that you can walk the mile in 20 minutes. Then, increase the distance to 1½ or 2 miles, three times per week. Invest in good walking shoes.

You can't afford to become sedentary; you'll gain weight, become depressed, and lose hope. You must commit yourself to exercise, no matter how non-physical it may seem.

As you become accustomed to walking, carry light weights in each hand, swinging your hands as you walk. Not only will you feel better emotionally and physically, but guess what? You will actually look forward to your walking sessions. I have found this to be a great time to spend alone with my wife, away from the phone and kids. Also, it is a wonderful time to think about all the blessings you have, in spite of your pain.

Swimming is another excellent exercise. By swimming, I do not mean competitive, hard swimming. Rather, I mean getting into warm water, walking, treading water, swimming slowly just to mobilize the chemicals from the brain and exercise your sore muscles.

By swimming, I mean getting into warm water, walking, treading water, swimming slowly just to mobilize the chemicals from the brain and exercise your sore muscles.

When you feel better, bike riding is another good exercise. However, you must be in pretty good shape and not experiencing a tremendous amount of pain. Like walking, riding a bicycle will allow the release of endorphins as natural pain killers.

One last exercise you might consider is low impact aerobics. Endorphins are released and yet you don't experience the hard jolts of high impact aerobics, which certainly can re-injure a TMJ.

Sleeping Position

The best position for sleeping is on your back. Unfortunately, most of us sleep on one side or another, or worse, on our stomachs. Sleeping on your back allows the muscles of the face and neck to relax. Sleeping on your side or stomach usually pushes your jaw to one side or the other, potentially causing further TMJ injury.

Place a small rolled towel or a small pillow behind your neck when you lie down. Also, place a pillow or a rolled bath towel behind your knees. This gives a slight bend in your legs and provides comfort to your lower back. If you must sleep on your side, bend your knees and place a pillow between them.

Acupressure

You may detect trigger points in your upper back, neck or jaw muscles but for any number of reasons, can't get to the doctor or therapist for treatment. Wouldn't it be nice to be able to treat some of them yourself? Well, you can, with help from a friend.

Acupressure is used to treat many trigger points. The technique consists of isolating trigger points, pressure on the trigger point, and massage of the area.

First, find the trigger point by localizing tender areas in muscles. You will feel the contracted area of the muscle: it will feel like a tiny BB below the skin. When compressed, a trigger point will be painful and may even refer pain to another area.

Have your spouse or friend firmly compress this area with their thumb. It will be painful for a few seconds. After 60 to 90 seconds, the pain will subside. This and the surrounding area should then be massaged for several seconds. Place a moist hot towel over the area for about 5 minutes. Then, remove the towel, compress the area and if a trigger point is found again, repeat the procedure.

Placing moist heat over the area or taking a hot shower just prior to applying pressure on the trigger points makes this procedure more effective. Expect soreness in the muscles; however, the next day the pain will be reduced.

Tennis ball therapy

Another technique to break up trigger points in your neck, shoulders, or upper back requires a tennis ball. Place a tennis ball on the floor and lie down, positioning the ball under the tender area. Move around slowly, using the ball to apply pressure to the trigger point. This breaks up the trigger point and reduces muscle pain.

Even if you're careful, there is a chance that your jaw will lock. This is especially true if you have a history of joint clicking or locking.

Apply heat over the painful area once the pain begins to subside. Repeat if the pain persists.

If Your Jaw Locks

Even if you're careful, even if you eat the proper foods and don't open your mouth for long periods of time, there is a chance that your jaw will lock. This is especially true if you have a history of joint clicking or locking. Locking can be of two types: open and closed.

Open locking

Yawning or wide opening to eat an apple or submarine sandwich may cause an open lock of the TMJ. If this happens, you will not be able to close your mouth. You'll be terrified the first time this occurs. However, this type of lock is easily reduced (unlocked). First, RELAX! If you can relax, the muscles may allow the jaw to close automatically. If not, try to push down and forward on your lower back teeth, using a quick jerk. Usually, this needs only to be done once.

If the joint still is locked, repeat this maneuver. If you are unsuccessful in unlocking your joints, then try to get help from a family member or neighbor or better yet, get to your dentist as quickly as possible.

If this happens on the weekend or after hours and you can't get hold of your dentist, you may have to go to an emergency room.

Yawning or wide opening to eat an apple may cause an open lock of the TMJ. If this happens, you will not be able to close your mouth. First, RELAX! If you can relax, the muscles may allow the jaw to close automatically.

After reduction of the open lock, apply icebags over both joints immediately and start taking aspirin, ibuprofen, or acetaminophen.

Closed locking

If you experience an inability to open your mouth, you either have a problem with the muscles that open the mouth, or the disc in one or both temporomandibular joints is out of place.

Muscle soreness. If the muscles are sore and irritated from bruxing, clenching, or an injury to the jaw, then apply moist heat to the joints or get into the shower and let the heat from the water penetrate the muscles around your TMJs. Then, slowly try to open. You may have to carefully pull on your lower jaw.

Once the jaw opens, apply ice over the joints and take aspirin or acetaminophen. Keep the jaw moving; don't stop even if the muscles are sore. Call your dentist and report this problem. He or she may refer you for physical therapy or chiropractic evaluation.

Displaced disc. The second cause of closed locking of the joints, a displaced disc, may or may not be painful. Usually, you will be able to open your mouth just about an inch. You might even be able to open wider if you gently move your jaw to one side or the other. If the disc is out of place, it will act like a stone caught between a door and the floor. Opening may be possible but difficult.

It's important to remember not to force your mouth open. You may cause further damage to the joints. Try to relax, open slowly, and then move your jaw back and forth slowly, trying to open after moving a few times. Usually, a "pop" will be heard when the disc goes back into place, and then you'll be able to open wide. However, if you close, the joints may lock again. Again, apply ice over the joints and begin taking aspirin, ibuprofen, or acetaminophen.

If either type of locking occurs again, you should see a TMJ specialist for treatment. Both of these problems respond well to splint therapy. The doctor may also order physical therapy, prescribe medications, and place you on a soft diet.

Twelve

Medications

Whether you have a TMJ problem or pain in another area of your body, you need to understand which medications are helpful and how they work.

The term *over-the-counter* simply means nonprescription medication. Aspirin or certain cold remedies are good examples of OTC medications. Even though a prescription isn't necessary, these drugs are very effective and when used properly, are quite safe. Drugs that reduce pain are termed analgesics.

Names

All medications have three names:

1. A *chemical* (scientific) name
2. A *trade* (proprietary) name
3. A *generic* (common) name

The scientific name is used by biochemists and doctors so that they can communicate no matter what the common name is. Generic names are easier to pronounce and remember. For example, if I told you to take acetylsalicylic acid (chemical name), you probably wouldn't have a clue. However, if I told you to take Bufferin (trade name), you would immediately understand that I was telling you to take aspirin (generic name).

NSAIDs

Aspirin and ibuprofen are classified as non-steroidal antiinflammatory drugs (NSAIDs). Both work within the central nervous system to reduce fever and at the site of injury to reduce inflammation, swelling and pain.

Medications are devised to work most efficiently when taken at specific times. If you don't take medication as recommended, then the blood levels begin to fall too much, thus reducing the effectiveness.

When tissue is injured, several complex chemical reactions take place which, if interrupted, don't produce the classic symptoms of swelling, pain, redness and heat. NSAIDs interrupt these chemical reactions, preventing the formation of pain-producing chemicals called prostaglandins. That's why it is so important to take NSAIDs as recommended, usually ever six hours. This orderly routine keeps the level of the chemical circulating at an effective level in the blood stream.

NSAIDs are often combined with other chemicals for specific results. For example, aspirin combined with an antacid is called buffered aspirin (one brand is Bufferin). Another NSAID compound, APC, is a combination of aspirin, phenacetin and caffeine.

If you're prescribed a stronger pain killer, you can improve the drug's effect by taking a couple aspirin or Tylenol with the medication, thus improving the desired effects without increasing the side-effects of the stronger drug. (**But check with your doctor before doing so.** Some prescribed medications already contain one of these ingredients, so you could overdose yourself.) Also be careful about increasing your dosage of drugs such as Tylenol #3. It is easy to reach toxic levels of the Tylenol.

Two other NSAIDs frequently used are Naprosyn and Daypro. These medications are effective in reducing both pain and inflammation when taken as prescribed.

This is an important point to understand. Medications, all types and not just analgesics, have been devised to work most efficiently when taken at specific times. For example, most analgesics work best when taken every 6 hours. If you don't take medication as recommended, then the blood levels begin to fall too much, thus reducing the effectiveness. This is so important that I can't stress it enough.

As was mentioned above, NSAIDs reduce pain AND inflammation. If you don't take these medications as recommended, the chemicals that produce inflammation will accumulate, causing further pain and swelling.

A few other examples of NSAIDs are Feldene, Orudis, Ansaid, Toradol, Tolectin, Relafin, and Lodine. As you can see, this inventory of NSAIDs is quite extensive, and not even a complete list. These medications are used for a variety of diseases with one common thread: all stop the chemical development of inflammation.

Although not classified as an NSAID, a new and very effective analgesic named *Ultram* may be a "wonder drug" for some. It has the strength of many prescription narcotics without their harmful effects. Better yet, Ultram can be used in combination with other pain medications to improve pain reduction without producing unwanted side effects. This medication, unfortunately, doesn't work for everyone and initially produces dizziness in about a third of those taking it.

Narcotics

Narcotics are the most effective pain killers, but they are addictive. Often, narcotics are mixed with aspirin or acetaminophen to increase the potency of the drug without increasing the amount of narcotic. For example, Empirin Compound with Codeine, Fiorinal with Codeine or Lorcet are examples of such mixtures. Darvon and Darvocet are similar medications but are classified as synthetic narcotics.

The major complication with these drugs, aside from the addictive possibilities, is depression of respiration. In other words, these drugs can slow or even stop breathing if taken in large quantities, especially when one is consuming alcohol. In addition, constipation, drowsiness, and stomach problems are frequent side-effects of narcotics.

Cortisone

Cortisone (also known as a corticosteroid) is an antiinflammatory medication that may be prescribed for any number of TMJ-related problems. However, due to side-effects, cortisone should be used sparingly. Taking cortisone pills for long periods of time can cause weight gain and can damage the liver and kidneys.

Cortisone may also be injected into the TMJ. This method of administration can cause damage to the bone and cartilage. However, there are times when cortisone is effective and necessary.

Local Anesthetics

Local anesthetics, often improperly called Novocaine, are used not only to anesthetize (numb) an area, but also for diagnostic and therapeutic purposes.

To diagnose a problem, local anesthetic injections are used to numb anatomical structures in an attempt to discover what, if any, structure or structures might be causing pain.

Local anesthetics are also used therapeutically to treat trigger points, or small spasms, in muscles. The anesthetic is injected directly into the trigger points to break up the spasms and produce relief by numbing the area. Local anesthetics may also be used in conjunction with cortisone to treat tendon, ligament and nerve injuries.

Muscle Relaxants

Another large and very important group of medications is muscle relaxants. These chemicals relax skeletal muscles, such as those in the head and neck regions. Relaxation of these muscles reduces or even relieves the formation of trigger points and therefore reduces pain. Examples of commonly prescribed muscle relaxants are Flexeril and Parafon Forte DSC.

The major side-effect of muscle relaxants is drowsiness and some stomach irritation. A newer medication, Skelaxin, works well to relax muscles but rarely produces sedation.

I often prescribe a muscle relaxant and ibuprofen together. In addition, I might refer the patient to a chiropractor or physical therapist, give trigger point injections, and place an intra-oral orthopedic appliance (discussed in Chapters 5 and 7). TMJ and muscle problems often need to be treated with many different modalities of treatment.

Antidepressants

The brain of people in pain frequently produces certain chemicals that, if reabsorbed by the brain, produce stimulation and interrupt normal sleep patterns.

Particular antidepressant medications are sometimes prescribed to prevent reabsorption of these chemicals. The most common is amitriptyline (generic name) or Elavil (brand or trade name). This drug, prescribed at bedtime, may produce water retention and drowsiness in the morning.

Another antidepressant is Desyrel and it too, is given at bedtime but may also produce drowsiness.

A new medication, Ambien, is also effective in the treatment of chronic pain but doesn't seem to produce the drowsiness of the other drugs. It too, is given at bedtime.

Table 21: Medications commonly used to treat TMJ**

Type of Drug	Brand Name	Generic Name	Desired Effects	Side Effects
Analgesic	Bufferin, Ascriptin, Anacin, Empirin, APC, Aspirin	Acetylsalicylic Acid (Aspirin)	Reduce inflammation, reduce pain, reduce fever	Stomach irritation and/or bleeding, reduce blood clotting
Analgesic	Tylenol, Datril, Anacin II	Acetaminophen	Reduce pain, reduce fever	Liver damage, glucose problems
Non-Opioid Analgesics (NSAIDs)	Ultram, Tramadol, Anaprox, Aleve, Naprosyn, Naprolen Toradol Lodine Relafin Dolabid Cataflam Daypro Ansaid Orudis Feldene Motrin, Advil	Naproxen sodium Ketorolac acid Etodolac acid Nabumetone Diflunisal Diclofenac Oxaprozin Flurbiprofen Ketoprofen Piroxicam Ibuprofen	Reduce pain, reduce fever, reduce inflammation	Stomach irritation, dizziness, interfere with calcium channel blockers (prolonged use)
Muscle Relaxants	Skelaxin Parafon forte DSC Flexeril Soma Norflex	Metaxalone Chlorzoxazone Cyclobenzaprine Carisoprodol Orphenadrine	Reduce muscle spasm	Drowsiness, stomach irritation
Anti-depressants	Desyrel Elavil Tofrinil	Trazodone Amitriptyline Imipramine	Improve sleep, reduce pain	Dry mouth, drowsiness
SSRI* Anti-depressants	Paxil Prozac Zoloft Effexor	Paroxetine HCl Fluoxetine HCl Sertraline HCl Venlafaxine	Improve sleep, decrease depression	Dry mouth, sexual dysfunction, drowsiness
Minor Tranquilizer	Valium Ativan Xanex	Diazepam Lorazepam Aloprazolam	Reduce muscle tension and anxiety	Drowsiness, addiction
Hypnotics	Ambien Restoril	Zolpidem Temazepam	Improve sleep	Drowsiness, headache, fatigue

* SSRI: Selective serotonin re-uptake inhibitor

** Naturopathic supplements and vitamins are discussed in Chapter 13.

Thirteen

Nutraceutical Support for TMJ

With Steve Fleshman, R.N., B.S.N., M.N.H., N.D. (candidate)

If you thought that the topic of TMJ was controversial, you haven't seen the field of nutrition!

Like most doctors (except chiropractors and naturopathic physicians), I was trained in traditional or allopathic nutrition. Although we had excellent training in biochemistry and physiology, our nutritional training was sadly lacking. It consisted of the four basic food groups and how to counsel our patients in the prevention of tooth decay and periodontal disease.

Body chemistry was not addressed. In fact, the concept of nutrition was scoffed. Medical science was far too advanced to worry about such trivial items as cellular metabolism and proper supplementation. Modern medicine had all the answers and besides, if we or our patients became ill, we'd just write a prescription and everything would be all right. Usually.

Enlightenment

When I was in my first year of dental school, I met my paternal grandfather, the late Dr. Earl Shankland of Cleveland, Ohio. At that time, he was in his middle 70s, healthy as a man half his age, and practicing dentistry five days a week.

The blessings of good health hadn't always been his. When he was in his early 60s, he had to retire from his beloved profession due to crippling arthritis of the hands and various other systemic diseases, all of which were considered normal for a 20th century American male. But my grandfather's life, and countless others which he'd influence later (including mine) was about to change when he read a little paperback book by one of those "odd-ball nutritionists:" *Let's Eat Right to Keep Fit*, written by Adele Davis.

My grandfather became the student of Ms. Davis, as well as a personal friend, and followed her recommendations religiously: no sugar; no bleached flour; wheat germ daily; and the use of antioxidant vitamins, especially vitamins C and E.

Within a matter of weeks my grandfather was no longer disabled. He resumed his dental practice, but practiced holistic, not allopathic, dentistry until well after his 87th birthday, working five days a week and even walking to his office when the streets were closed due to those famous heavy snows that Lake Erie frequently provides to that part of Ohio.

I was amazed at his knowledge of biochemistry and physiology. After spending some time in his office, I was mystified by patient after patient who told me stories about their failing health that only improved after my grandfather guided them into holistic medicine and good, science-based nutrition.

In 1975 he told me that one of the main causes of diabetes was a chromium deficiency, a scientific fact that only in the last few months has been accepted by the established scientific community! He changed the lives of many patients who thought they were doomed to a life of disability and suffering. His influence on the people of Cleveland is still felt today, nearly 10 years after his death.

What was I to do? My excellent training was unashamedly in allopathic medicine and yet, I knew there was more to nutrition than just the four basic food groups. After all, hadn't antibiotics saved countless lives? What about hypertensive medication? And what about the use of mercury in dental amalgams?

These and many other questions plagued me long after my formal training ended. I began experimenting with various combinations of minerals and vitamins and coupled these with allopathic medicine. I now incorporate both philosophies in my approach to TMJ problems, recognizing the tremendous biological variability among us human beings.

Getting Down to Basics

Below are a few concepts of nutrition that are not the all in all. There's so much more that I won't pretend to understand and I freely admit I can't present here. Study for yourself and think.

Don't automatically assume that any health care professional knows anything about proper nutrition. Most do not and in fact, will almost brag about a lack of nutritional knowledge.

Ask at health food stores which books they'd recommend studying and learn for yourself. After all, your health is your responsibility, not the doctor's.

Natural medicine has experienced a resurgence of interest from the health care community. Medical researchers now possess the technology and understanding to appreciate the value of "natural" therapies.

For example, the prestigious magazine *Nature* just reported that vitamin E appears to not only help prevent cancer, but also enhances the effectiveness of chemotherapy drugs used to treat colorectal cancer. This is a specific case among many natural therapies being improved or refined through scientific investigation. Naturopathy is paving the way for medicine of the future — a medicine that recognizes the **healing power of nature**.

As with other joints, it seems highly likely that the various TMJ disorders could respond very well to natural modalities of treatment. This is especially true with nutraceuticals, which have been helpful in the treatment of conditions similar to TMJ like osteoarthritis.

Before discussing nature's healing power as it pertains to TMJ, let's establish a few naturopathic principles.

Table 22: Naturopathic principles

Principle 1: Remember that your body was created with a considerable power to heal itself. The role of the physician or therapist or healer is to facilitate and enhance this marvelous healing process, preferably with the aid of natural, non-toxic therapies. As Hippocrates so wisely wrote in the oath that now bears his name: "The physician must do no harm."

Principle 2: View the whole person. An individual must be seen as a whole, composed of a complex interaction of body, mind and spirit.

Principle 3: Identify and treat the cause. It's important to discover the underlying cause of a disease or disorder rather than simply suppress the symptoms. Symptoms are expressions of the body's attempt to heal. Causes spring from the physical, mental, emotional, and physical levels of our complex being.

Principle 4: The physician, healer or therapist is but a teacher, striving to educate, empower, and motivate the patient to assume personal responsibility for his or her health. This requires the doctor him- or herself to have a healthy attitude, lifestyle, and diet.

Principle 5: Prevention is the best cure. Prevention of disease is best accomplished through dietary habits and a healthy lifestyle, both of which support health and prevent disease.

Realize that TMJ, like other chronic disorders, responds best when these five naturopathic philosophies are faithfully applied. These philosophies, like the Ten Commandments, are difficult to follow all the time. But like our Creator, our bodies are very forgiving.

A TMJ Nutraceutical Insurance Plan

Whether you have a TMJ problem or are blessed with good health, the overwhelming scientific evidence supports the benefits of a "nutraceutical insurance plan." Remember that treating a chronic medical condition involves more than just haphazardly swallowing a handful of pills.

Michael Murray, N.D., in his authoritative and comprehensive book, *Encyclopedia of Nutritional Supplements,* recommends the following:

1. **Take a high quality vitamin and mineral supplement.** The sad truth is you get what you pay for. Have you heard the saying, "Don't take chances with parachute packers or your health?"

2. **Take extra antioxidants.** Hardly a week passes that the press doesn't report another scientific study recommending the use of antioxidants. Science is finally catching up with naturopathy.

3. **Take one tablespoon of flaxseed oil daily.** This natural oil is an excellent source of omega 3 fatty acids. Among its other benefits, it reduces the production of arachidonic acid, the precursor of many inflammatory products that are the chief causes of inflammation and localized pain.

TMJ and other joint problems may respond to the use of chondroitin sulfate and glucosamine. These nutrients are building blocks for cartilage formation during healing. (See below.)

Remember, it takes time to notice the effects of these and other nutraceuticals. Do not expect immediate results or else you'll be sorely disappointed. After all, your TMJ degeneration did not take place overnight, and will require some time to heal.

The following charts give recommended dosages for various nutraceuticals. Remember, dosages should be individualized for each person.

Table 23: Nutraceutical recommendations

Vitamin	Range for Adults (daily doses)	Comments
Vitamin A (Retinol)	5,000 IU*	Women of child-bearing age should not take more than 2,500 IU per day due to the possible risk of birth defects should they become pregnant
Vitamin A (from beta carotene)	5,000 - 25,000 IU	Mixed carotenoids are best
Vitamin D	100 - 400 IU	Nursing home patients in northern latitudes should have the high dose
Vitamin E (d-alpha tocopherol)	100 - 800 IU	Mixed tocopherols are best
Vitamin K (phytonadione)	60 - 300 mcg**	Essential in blood clotting
Vitamin C (ascorbic acid)	100 - 1,000 mg+	Divided doses in morning and evening
Vitamin B1 (thiamin)	10 - 100 mg	Essential for energy production, nerve function, and metabolism
Vitamin B 2 (riboflavin)	10 - 50 mg	Coenzyme in energy production
Vitamin B12 (Cobalamin)	400 mcg	Used in the synthesis of DNA, red blood cells and nerve cell insulation
Vitamin B 3 (Niacin)	10 - 100 mg	Essential for energy production, blood sugar regulation, antioxidant mechanisms, detoxification reactions; fat metabolism
Vitamin B6 (pyridoxine)	25 - 100 mg	Formation of body's protein structure; neurotransmitter; hormone balance
Biotin	100 - 300 mcg	Coenzyme in 4 enzymes; metabolism of sugars, fats and amino acids
Pantothenic acid	25 - 100 mg	Needed in synthesis of acetyl-coenzyme A; important for synthesis of red blood cells and adrenal hormones
Folic acid	400 mcg	Works with Vit B12 in many reactions; critical for normal cellular division (DNA synthesis) & nervous system development
Choline	10 - 100 mg	Critical for synthesis of neurotransmitters and many components of cell membranes; important in metabolism of fats
Inositol	10 - 100 mg	"Unofficial" Vit B; used in cellular membrane reactions

*IU-International units **mcg-micrograms +mg-milligrams

Table 24: Recommended daily minerals

Minerals	Adult Range	Comments
Boron	1 - 6 mg	Functions in normal bone and joint health; deficiency may be linked to postmenopausal bone loss
Calcium	250 - 1,250 mg	Most abundant mineral in the body; functions in maintenance of healthy bones and many enzyme reactions; woman at risk for or suffering from osteoporosis may need to take a separate calcium supplement when trying to achieve higher dosage levels
Chromium	200 - 400 mcg	For diabetes and weight loss, dosages of 600 mcg (consult with physician if you're diabetic)
Copper	1 -2 mg	Needed in collagen formation and many other enzyme reactions
Iodine	50 - 150 mcg	Important in normal thyroid function; may modulate the effect of estrogen on breast tissue
Iron	15 - 30 mg	Men and post-menopausal women rarely need supplemental iron
Magnesium	250 - 500 mg	When magnesium therapy is indicated, take a separate magnesium supplement
Manganese	10 - 15 mg	Functions in many enzyme systems, especially those involved with blood sugar control, energy metabolism, thyroid function and antioxidant reactions
Molybdenum	10 - 25 mcg	Coenzyme for xanthine oxidase, aldehyde oxidase, and sulfate oxidase
Potassium	200 - 500 mg	Important for normal nerve function
Selenium	100 - 200 mcg	Important as an antioxidant and in miroctubule formation
Silica	1 - 25 mg	Essential for healthy hair and nails
Vanadium	50 - 100 mcg	Improves mineralization of bone and teeth; may have a role in insulin and cholesterol regulation
Zinc	15 - 45 mg	Component of over 200 enzymes; needed for proper function of many hormones

Table 25: Daily antioxidant recommendations

Antioxidant	Daily Dosage	Comments
Vitamin E (d-alpha tocopherol)	400 - 800 IU	Mixed tocopherols offer greater coverage
Vitamin C (ascorbic acid)	500 - 1,500 mg	Consider Ester C
Flaxseed Oil	One tablespoon	Also available in capsules

Essential fatty acids

Experts estimate that approximately 80% of our population consume an insufficient amount of essential fatty acids. In addition to playing a critical role in normal cellular physiology, essential fatty acids reduce and actually reverse heart disease, cancer, autoimmune diseases (for example, multiple sclerosis and rheumatoid arthritis), and many skin diseases. Research indicates that over 60 health conditions benefit from essential fatty acid supplementation.

Although degeneration of the articular surfaces of the TMJ is anatomically unique, remember that the TMJ is still a joint, like the knee or elbow. Many therapies for other joints apply very nicely in treating the TMJ.

Herbs

The use of herbs to treat TMJ problems is gaining acceptance among even the most traditional allopathic doctors. Such natural products as blue violet, catnip, chamomile, hops, lobelia, skullcap, kava, thyme, red raspberry, passion flower, valerian root and wild lettuce have calming and anti-stress properties. Take these as directed on the labels. Experiment with each or combinations of each to suit your needs in the overall treatment of your TMJ problems. Consult with a naturopath or inquire at a natural health food store if you need more information.

Table 26: Recommended daily supplementation for TMJ

Supplement	Suggested Daily Dosage	Comments
Calcium*	2,000 mg	For proper muscular function and calming. Prevents decalcification of bone and relieves stress. Use chelated forms
Magnesium*	1,500 mg in divided dosages: after meals and at bedtime	For proper muscle function
Vitamin B Complex*	100 mg 3 times/day	Provides all the benefits of the B vitamins
Pantothenic acid*	100 mg twice a day	Participates in release of energy from fats, carbohydrates & proteins; improves body's resistence to stress
Coenzyme Q10+	10 mg	Improves oxygenation of tissues
L-tyrosine+	500 mg at bedtime on empty stomach with water or juice, NOT milk. For better absorption, take with 500 mg Vitamin C	Improves quality of sleep and relieves anxiety and reduces depression. Caution: do not take tyrosine if you're taking an MAO inhibitor drug
Multivitamins & minerals complex+	As directed	For balanced nutrients
Vitamin C+	4,000 - 8,000 mg	Combats stress and is necessary in adrenal gland function. Also, a coenzyme in the repair in production of collagen

* Essential + Helpful

Don't use chamomile regularly because you could develop a ragweed allergy. Avoid chamomile totally if you know that you're allergic to ragweed. Don't take lobelia internally for a long period of time.

Arthritis Cure?

Once the bony surfaces of any synovial joint are injured, osteoarthritis will develop. This damage, at first, is chiefly due to the cartilage on the bony surfaces of joints.

In the temporomandibular joint, such symptoms as joint pain and swelling, the feeling of heat over the joint and crunching sounds (termed crepitus) indicate that osteoarthritis (or degenerative joint disease) is present. Unfortunately, osteoarthritis may cause such constant and intense pain that many with this rather common disorder undergo surgery, only to have the problem worsen.

In Europe (and for many years in the United States in veterinary medicine), two natural chemicals have been used very effectively to actually cause *growth of new cartilage with reduction of the symptoms of osteoarthritis.* According to Drs. Theodosakis and Adderly, in *The Arthritis Cure*, chondroitin sulfate and glucosamine in combination with vitamin C and manganese have been extremely helpful in treating osteoarthritis. I too, have discovered this to be true in treating patients with osteoarthritis of the TMJ.

Glucosamine

The body manufactures glucosamine. This molecule is composed of a glucose (table sugar) and an amine (a nitrogen and two molecules of hydrogen from the amino acid glutamine). Its physiological function is to stimulate the synthesis of substances needed for normal synovial joint function and for stimulating cartilage repair in joints. Also, the molecule itself is *hydrophilic* (water loving) and actually soaks up water into the cartilage matrix, thus increasing elasticity and improving the spongy quality of cartilage.

It seems that as we normally age, we lose the ability to produce adequate quantities of glucosamine. This causes cartilage to lose its elasticity and ability to repair itself. If arthritis begins, as it often does in a damaged TMJ in middle age, the cartilage can't repair itself. Swelling and joint pain soon begin as the joint surfaces deteriorate.

Chondroitin sulfate

Chondroitin sulfate is also very useful in improving the function of cartilage. This compound was originally present in our bodies when we formed the cartilage in our joints and when the bones of our skulls formed, but as we age, it too diminishes in concentration. Chondroitin sulfate molecular chains, like glucosamine, have negative electrical charges that are hydrophilic. They greatly attract water molecules, and like glucosamine, incorporate water into the molecular chains.

When a joint is resting, the glucosamine and chondroitin sulfate molecules attract water into the synovial fluid. When the cartilage is under function and squeezed, the water is squeezed out. Since cartilage has no blood supply itself, this incorporation of water and synovial fluid provides nourishment to the cartilage and removes waste products.

Repeated joint stress (even when associated with normal function) can, in the presence of an injury or pathological condition, weaken or damage the cartilage. Cartilage repair is very slow at best due to its poor nutrient supply and because the joint rarely rests.

Glucosamine and chondroitin sulfate are essential to the repair and growth of cartilage. The production of these molecules diminishes with age, stress or joint injury.

Taken in conjunction with glucosamine sulfate, vitamin C and manganese, chondroitin sulfate aids in the repair of joint cartilage, possibly by the reformation of new cartilage and the reduction of inflammation. This in itself reduces joint pain and swelling.

Taken together, glucosamine improves the body's absorption of chondroitin sulfate. And what's really important and interesting is that when taken up by existing cartilage, glucosamine *stimulates the production of chondroitin sulfate within cartilage*. These processes are important in production of new cartilage and repair of the existing damaged cartilage.

Go to any health food store, or where supplements are sold, and purchase these two natural products. Take them in the following manner in divided doses:

Table 27: Determining dosage level

Your Weight	**Dosages of Supplements**
Less than 120 lbs	1. 1,000 mg glucosamine 2. 800 to 1000 mg chondroitin sulfate 3. 1,000 to 2,000 mg Vit C 4. 25mg manganese
Between 120 and 200 lbs	1. 1,500 mg glucosamine 2. 1,200 mg chondroitin sulfate 3. 3,000 to 4,000 mg Vit C 4. 25 to 50 mg manganese
Over 200 lbs	1. 2,000 mg glucosamine 2. 1,600 mg chondroitin sulfate 3. 3,000 to 4,000 mg Vit C 4. 50 mg manganese

Modified after: Theodosakis J and Adderly B. *The Arthritis Cure.* New York: St. Martin's Press; 1997:76.

Use these doses as approximate values and experiment with them. I've found that my patients report a noticeable improvement in the symptoms of osteoarthritis in about two to four weeks. Vitamin C and manganese, which serve as coenzymes in the synthesis of cartilage, also function as antioxidants. So, taking vitamin C and manganese you receive benefits far greater than cartilage formation. As with all supplements, these dosages vary from person to person.

What about side effects? The main side effects, especially of glucosamine, are stomach upset, heartburn, diarrhea, and indigestion. If you develop these symptoms, take these nutraceuticals with meals. As of now, no allergic reactions to glucosamine or chondroitin sulfate have been reported.

A Good Night's Sleep

Remember in Chapter 12 when we discussed the use of certain antidepressants to help chronic pain patients sleep better? How would you like the same benefits without the side effects?

The hormone melatonin is produced in our pineal gland but only during darkness. In fact, its production is inhibited by light. It's a very powerful antioxidant, able to permeate every cell in the body. It specifically protects DNA and aids in repair of the nuclear material in the cell.

More importantly for the chronic pain patient, melatonin provides sedative properties, helping to reduce anxiety, panic disorders, and inducing sleep. It appears that this hormone may be one of the chief regulators of our internal body clock. But like so many other hormones, the production of melatonin falls as we age. Therefore, we may need to take supplements of melatonin.

There is no established dose for melatonin, so you'll have to experiment to find your ideal dose. Some people take a very small amount and find good results. Others have to gradually increase the dosage to reach their optimal level.

If you decide to try melatonin (after discussing this with your doctor), start by taking ½ of a milligram about an hour before bedtime. If you still don't sleep well, keep adding increments of ½ milligram every few nights up to around 3 milligrams or so. You'll sleep soundly, going through all the important stages of sleep just as if you'd taken amitriptyline, but without the side effects of drowsiness and weight gain.

Remember, it's vitally important for TMJ sufferers to be able to sleep well, and melatonin can help. I am using it more and more in my practice with good results for my patients. You'll find melatonin especially helpful if you have to work irregular hours or if you travel between time zones.

As with all medications and nutraceuticals, pregnant women and nursing mothers should consult their physician before taking melatonin. But rest assured, melatonin has been found very safe, with only two main side effects: (1) providing no *noticeable* effects whatsoever, and (2) drowsiness for the first few mornings after its initial use.

Fourteen

Finding Help

Finding a TMJ doctor may be more difficult than one would believe. Some physicians (dentists, medical doctors, psychologists) doubt that TMJ exists.

Most don't deny TMJ problems but doubt that so many people can be affected by a disorder that until recently, wasn't even discussed or taught. Other doctors believe that TMJ clicking can signify a dislocation and a cause of pain but don't recognize any other disorder such as temporal tendinitis or Ernest syndrome. Still others propose that the only treatment necessary for TMJ problems is medication, rest and psychological consultation. Yet another group feels that no treatment is needed, but those at the other end of the spectrum prescribe only surgery if medications don't work.

What can you, as the patient and consumer, do to find the proper type of therapist? How can you be sure the doctor you consult knows anything about TMJ? In my opinion, these are some of the reasons why the cost of the treatment of head and TMJ pain is appears to be so high. By the time you find someone who can treat you effectively, chances are you have seen several doctors with little or no results.

What's the answer? First, understand that medical doctors have a hard time believing that a temporomandibular disorder could cause so much pain or produce so many problems. Most likely, they were taught nothing about TMJ in medical school or postgraduate training. They have a difficult time understanding the influence the TMJs exert on the upper body.

Unfortunately, medical doctors usually diagnose TMJ pain as migraine or sinus problems. When the patient doesn't respond to traditional therapy for these disorders, the doctor is likely to refer them to an ENT physician, a neurologist and ultimately, a psychiatrist.

Even though doctors believe that TMJ disorders exist, they often look only at the joint and not at other structures. This is especially true in the case of Ernest syndrome, temporal tendinitis, and occipital neuralgia.

Many oral and maxillofacial surgeons, on the other hand, deny the devastating effects that many TMJ problems have on the sufferer. These dentists (who have a residency in surgery after dental school) generally believe in the "Psychophysiologic Theory of Pain." This theory, first popularized in 1969 by oral surgeon Dr. Daniel Laskin, maintains that TMJ problems can be treated with medication and psychological counseling and usually, nothing else.

This theory also proposes that nearly all TMJ problems are produced by stress in the sufferer's life and that elimination of the stress will eliminate the TMJ problem. This theory has been prominent in the training of most oral surgeons. This is another reason why consulting an oral and maxillofacial surgeon initially may not be wise.

However, many if not most general practitioners of dentistry provide much more help or support than do oral surgeons. This certainly seems odd and sad. If it weren't for a few pioneers in dentistry, the diagnosis and treatment of TMJ problems would be worse than they presently are.

Why such diversity in dentistry? First we must consider the type of education in dental school. Most professors of dentistry in the United States, Canada and the rest of the Western world don't practice; they teach only and unfortunately, they teach as they were taught. Therefore, if these well-meaning professors never learned about TMJ problems, they couldn't possibly teach dental students or residents.

Second, treatment varies throughout the U.S. Although treatment modalities are becoming more consistent and recognized, there still is a great diversity. (Of course, diversity is not always wrong. There may be different ways to treat the same TMJ problem.)

Third, even though doctors (dentists, primarily) believe that TMJ disorders exist, they often look only at the joint and not at other structures. This is especially true in the case of Ernest syndrome, temporal tendinitis, and occipital neuralgia. These disorders have only in recent years been discovered and described in the scientific literature. Unfortunately, doctors haven't had the opportunity to read all the journal papers because there are so many journals. I estimate that it will take at least one entire generation of dentists before recognition of these other disorders becomes common.

It is amazing that insurance companies provide benefits for all joints except the TMJ. Because of the headaches caused by insurance companies, many doctors refuse to treat TMJ problems.

Fourth, many dentists don't treat TMJ problems because of poor insurance coverage. It is amazing that insurance companies will provide benefits for all other joints except the TMJ. Therefore, and due to the headaches (no pun intended!) caused by insurance companies, many doctors simply refuse to treat TMJ problems. As time goes by, these frustrated practitioners forget to even ask patients if they have symptoms of TMJ. The patient is the true victim of these administrative disputes.

There is no TMJ specialty in dentistry at the present time. Unlike medicine, there are only eight recognized dental specialties (endodontics, oral and maxillofacial surgery, prosthodontics, periodontics, orthodontics, oral pathology, pedodontics, and public health).

However, the American Academy of Head, Neck & Facial Pain and the American Academy of Orofacial Pain are currently working with the American Dental Association to establish a specialty of Orofacial Pain (the actual name of such a proposed specialty has not been determined yet). We're optimistic that the House of Delegates of the ADA will soon approve our application and establish such a specialty.

Until then, you, the patient and consumer, will have to search for a doctor who has training and experience in the diagnosis and treatment of TMJ and related disorders. I suggest that you use Appendix A as a guide.

Thus far, I haven't given you the answer as to how to can find a competent TMJ doctor. As you can surmise, this is somewhat difficult. However, there are a few guidelines that you should follow.

Questions

When calling an office to make an appointment, ask the receptionist to give some information about the doctor.

Table 28: Questions to ask about a doctor

1. **Does he or she treat many TMJ patients?** Unfortunately, the doctor may be wonderful and quite knowledgeable but if few TMJ patients are treated in that office, do you really want to seek care there?

2. **From where do the patients come?** Although it is not always true or a requirement, but knowledgeable doctors treating TMJ generally have patients travel vast distances to see them. Again, this doesn't ensure quality or knowledge.

Table 28: Questions to ask about a doctor *(cont)*

3. **What kind of training has the doctor had** and does he or she attend seminars about TMJ and related problems? Avoid anyone who doesn't keep up to date in any area of medicine, especially TMJ.

4. **Does the doctor often recommend surgery?** In my practice, I see the worst of the worst patients and only approximately 1-2% of my patients ultimately require TMJ surgery. In my opinion, avoid any doctor recommending more surgery than 1-3% of his or her TMJ patients.

5. **Does the doctor recommend the use of splints?** It is impossible (and illegal) for the receptionist to diagnose your problems by phone; however, the American Dental Association, the American Academy of Head, Neck & Facial Pain, and the American Academy of Orofacial Pain all recommend the use of conservative, reversible initial treatment for TMJ. This generally means a splint.

6. **Does the doctor work with other doctors such as chiropractic physicians?** This is important; no doctor can be a Lone Ranger and know-it-all. If he or she claims such nonsense, get out of that office!

7. **Ask if the doctor would be offended if you asked for another doctor to give you a second opinion.** If a doctor is sure of his or her diagnosis and recommended treatment, a second opinion will be welcomed and not rejected.

8. **Ask if the doctor adjusts the teeth to treat TMJ.** If he or she does without first using conservative, reversible treatment (for example, a splint), then find another doctor.

9. **Ask if the doctor belongs to any TMJ academies or professional groups.**

Although membership in a professional group isn't mandatory to demonstrate that the doctor has knowledge concerning TMJ, most do belong to one or more of the following groups:

Table 29: Professional organizations for TMJ practitioners

A. The American Academy of Head, Neck & Facial Pain
B. The American Equilibration Society
C. The American Academy of Orofacial Pain (formerly, the American Academy of Craniomandibular Disorders)
D. The International College of Craniomandibular Orthopedics

At your appointment, as the doctor interviews you, interview him or her. Unless you are geographically isolated, allow this doctor to treat you only if you trust and can communicate with him or her. Wouldn't you do the same with a mechanic or builder?

Also, don't engage in treatment until you understand what the risks of treatment, of no treatment and of alternative treatments. Not all TMJ problems need to be treated with more than a soft diet, moist heat and over-the-counter medications from time to time. Not all knee or elbow injuries are treated. So, why would all TMJ problems need treatment as well?

Further, make certain that you understand what treatment the doctor recommends. In fact, ask for a written statement concerning the proposed treatment and its cost. Ask what time frame the doctor is thinking and when you might begin to see improvement.

Remember that even though you must rely upon someone to treat your TMJ problem, understand that they are working for you. I know that this is not a traditional way to view health care. Yet, why should these services be different than any other type of service you may need? Don't allow someone to recommend, much less perform, any type of treatment that doesn't sound right. If the doctor makes a recommendation that you don't feel comfortable with, then ask him or her if there are alternatives. Perhaps there will be none; however, that is rare.

Fifteen

The NTI

Necessity as the Mother of Ingenuity

Just when everyone thought that the controversies concerning splints were settled (well, kind of), new information surfaced that has shaken the foundations of dentistry and medicine. A migraine sufferer (who also happened to be a dentist who works with TMJ patients) made a revolutionary discovery.

Dr. James Boyd suffered daily, *all day* headaches for over 12 years. The last five of those years, he had worn a traditional splint like that described in Chapter Five. His TMJ symptoms of joint popping and soreness were relieved, but his headaches persisted.

Like all of us who treat TMJ patients, Dr. Boyd was keenly aware of those patients who didn't respond to splint therapy. What he discovered was that some patients, including himself, were *primary clenchers*, whereas most others were *chronic bruxers*. Chronic bruxers, who clench their teeth together uncontrollably, also grind their teeth left, right and forward, wearing characteristic patterns into their teeth.

By contrast, primary clenchers suffer with headaches and sore neck muscles (classic TMJ symptoms), but they seem not to have wear patterns in their teeth and often don't suffer with TMJ pain.

Realizing that he was a primary clencher, Dr. Boyd modified his existing flat-plane splint, but wasn't comfortable until he adjusted the splint so that it touched at only one point in the front. However, when he would move his lower jaw around, the back portion of the splint would contact his lower teeth, and his headache returned. Using this information, Dr. Boyd invented the splint that he has named the *Nociceptive Trigeminal Inhibition* appliance, or *NTI*.

Research Supports the NTI

Neuroscientists know that clenching of the teeth involves contraction of the temporalis muscles, causing little or no tooth wear. However, the activity of bruxism requires that the temporalis muscles contract *along with* the lateral pterygoid muscles, which move the mandible left and right, producing a grinding effect and subsequent tooth wear, tooth sensitivity, and even loose teeth.

Continual contraction of the temporalis muscle (in other words, clenching) can cause muscle contraction or tension headaches in non-TMJ patients. These patients habitually clench their teeth, especially while sleeping. The temporalis muscles become fatigued, most likely due to a build-up of lactic acid and a decrease in oxygen in the muscles. The muscles go into spasm and a headache develops.

The traditional flat plane splint may even perpetuate temporalis muscle activity, *intensifying* the conditions for the severe headache sufferer. These are the patients who suffer with chronic headaches, sore necks, and even TMJ-like symptoms, but fail to respond to TMJ treatment. I suspect that far too many of these patients have endured unnecessary and debilitating TMJ surgery — or multiple surgeries.

Intense bruxing, a combination of grinding and clenching, causes tension headaches, especially in those who have TMJ problems. Unlike primary clenchers, these patients respond well to flat plane splint therapy.

How the NTI Works

Primary clenchers squeeze their teeth quite forcefully. A person may clench as much as 60% of his or her maximum voluntary clenching force. Some people might even clench harder when asleep than they can when asked to bite down as hard as they can! This maximal clenching force far exceeds any forces used for chewing.

The NTI seems to work by *suppressing the intensity of temporalis contraction* (clenching) to a level less than the threshold needed to create painful muscle symptoms. This acrylic appliance (Figures 24, 25 and 26) is placed on the upper front teeth and provides a pin-point contact with one or two (at the most) lower front teeth when biting up and moving the mandible laterally.

This modification produces a major neurological effect: the temporalis muscles relax due to the *inhibition* of certain trigeminal nerve reflexes. Hence, the name: Nociceptive Trigeminal Inhibition (NTI) appliance.

The NTI is worn only when sleeping. By taking the NTI appliance out of the mouth when chewing, the back teeth are stimulated and therefore don't move out of their normal jaw positions. (This is one of the major problems with other anterior bite planes that are used for TMJ treatment.) But because the NTI appliance is worn only a few hours while sleeping, the back teeth don't migrate.

The Really Exciting News about the NTI

If the NTI appliance only reduced tension-type headaches, that would be enough. In fact, the U.S. Food and Drug Administration has already approved the NTI for "the prevention of chronic tension and TMJ syndrome." (It's very unusual for the FDA to give such a recommendation to a device and allow the claim of "prevention" of a disorder.)

But what about migraine headaches? As mentioned in Chapter 8, migraines can debilitate people for up to 36 hours. Migraines occur in over

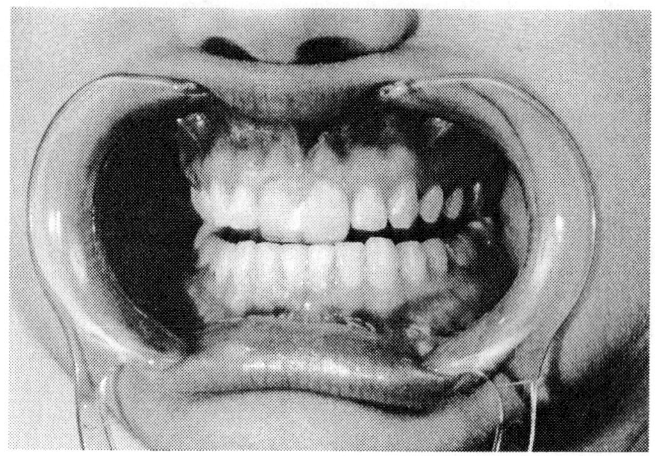

Figure 24: Daytime NTI appliance

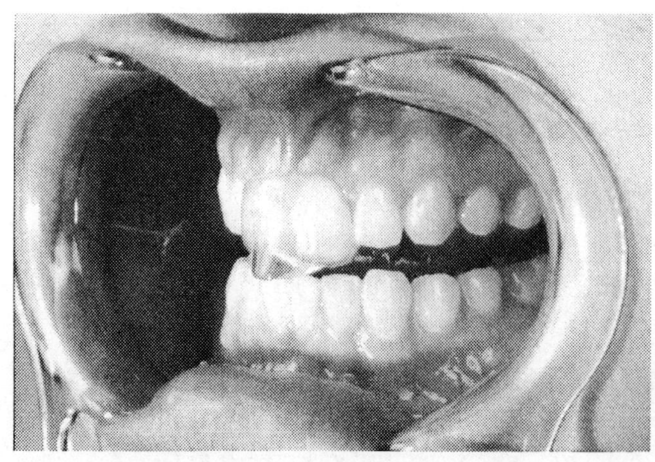

Figure 25: Nighttime NTI appliance

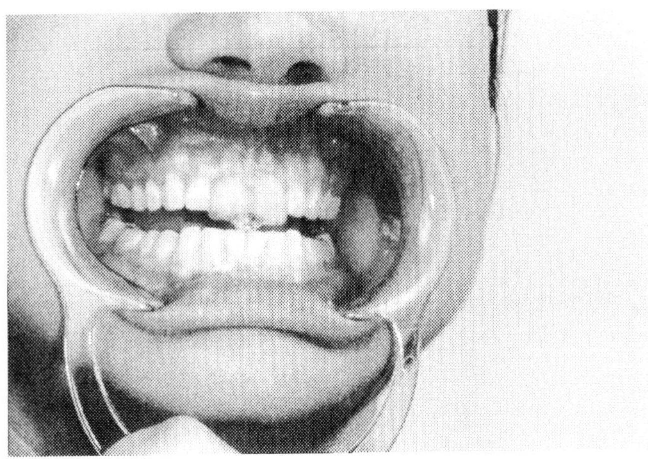

Figure 26: Close-up, NTI night appliance

45 million people in the United States alone! Billions of work-dollars are lost annually due to these terrible headaches.

There are many different theories about the cause of migraines. Neuro-chemicals (and perhaps chemicals traveling through the blood) are common factors in all migraine theories. Epinephrine (adrenaline) is one good example. Whenever you're upset and stressed, epinephrine is released from the cortical area of your adrenal glands, preparing you for the classic "fight or flight" reaction. If your epinephrine levels are elevated due to the stresses of everyday life and you tend to clench your teeth, you'll bite down hard when sleeping, chronically tensing your temporalis muscles.

Clenching has been implicated as one cause of migraine headaches, or at least a cause for the painful complications of migraine. Again, primary clenching, not bruxing, produces the increased temporalis muscle tightening or contraction. Many researchers feel that such tightening of the temporalis muscle is a major physical cause of migraine headache, and the NTI produces *relaxation* of the temporalis muscles. The NTI may also work because it slightly increases the space between the teeth (called "the vertical dimension" by dentists) and this, too, seems to relax the temporalis muscles.

That's why the NTI is so effective! This appliance reduces temporalis muscle contraction and migraine headaches in approximately 56% to 91% of migraine patients as demonstrated in three separate studies. In addition, the NTI reduces the maximum clenching force of the teeth by over two-thirds of that of patients wearing no appliance at all; this finding alone is known to reduce migraine headaches.

At the time of this writing, the NTI can't legally be called a *migraine-treating* appliance, although it seems as if it is. Current FDA studies should soon prove that the NTI does, in fact, *prevent and treat migraine headaches* in many migraineurs.

So What?

What am I trying to say? In brief, the NTI appears to be a revolutionary new oral appliance which has wonderful promise in not only treating but preventing migraine headaches in as many as 56% to 91% of migraine sufferers. These figures are amazing — no migraine medication to date can begin to boast of such high numbers. Best of all, the NTI is not a drug and there are no side effects.

You might wonder if your TMJ doctor or family dentist can treat you or a loved one for migraine and tension headaches with the NTI. The answer is yes, if the doctor has had training in the fabrication and use of the appliance. Your doctor may obtain information from the Heraeus Kulzer, Inc. (South Bend, IN), 219-291-0661, or the Headache Prevention Institute, 248-258-6182, about common migraine.

Appendix A

Resources

Professional Associations for TMJ Practitioners

1. **The American Academy of Head, Neck & Facial Pain.** 520 West Pipeline Road, Hurst, TX 76053. 1-(800)-322-TMJ1. This academy was formed in 1985 and is comprised primarily of dentists who treat TMJ problems.

   Web address: http://www.aahnfp.org

2. **The American Equilibration Society.** 8726 N. Ferris Avenue, Morton Grove, IL 60053. 1-(708)-965-2888. The AES was the first academy formed for doctors specifically dealing with TMJ problems. It is primarily composed of dentists and physical therapists.

   Web address: http://www.prosthodontics.org/aes

3. **The American Academy of Orofacial Pain.** 19 Mantua Rd., Mt. Royal, NJ 08061. 1-(609)-423-7222. The academy, formerly the American Academy of Craniomandibular Disorders, is comprised primarily of dentists who treat TMJ problems. Many of the members are academicians and professors in the U.S. and Canada.

   Web address: http://www.aaop.org

4. **TMJ & Stress Center.** P.O. Box 803394, Dallas, TX 75380. 1-(800)-533-5121. A support center for TMJ patients was founded by a TMJ sufferer. Her mission is to educate the public concerning TMJ.

   Web address: http://www.myodata.com

5. **The American Academy of Pain Management.** 3600 Sisk Road, Suite D, Modesto, CA 95356. 1-(209)-533-9744. Health care professionals of various backgrounds: dentistry, medicine, chiropractic, psychology, nursing and physical therapy.

   Web address: http://www.aapainmanage.org

6. **Headache Prevention Institute.** Dr. James Boyd, inventor of the NTI appliance. 1-(248)-258-6182.

   Web address: http://www.h-p-i.com

Affiliations

1. **American Association of Acupuncture and Oriental Medicine.** 4101 Lake Boone Trail, Suite 201, Raleigh, NC 27607. 1-(919)-787-5181. Provides referrals.

2. **American Association of Naturopathic Physicians.** 601 Valley, #105, Seattle WA 98109. 1-(206)-298-0126.

   http://www.naturopathic.org

3. **American Chronic Pain Association.** P.O. Box 850, Rocklin, CA 95677. 1-(916)-632-0922. The *ACPA Chronicle* is published quarterly, and includes articles, essays and book reviews written by people with chronic pain. This group also sponsors the ACPA Writing Connection, linking people through letters and phone calls.

4. **American Holistic Medical Association.** 2002 Eastlake Ave. E, Seattle, WA 98102. 1-(206)-322-6842. Can refer to members of this organization.

5. **American Nutritionists Association.** P.O. Box 34030, Bethesda, MD 20817. Members have advanced degrees in nutrition from accredited schools. Write to request a list of nutrition consultants; include a self-addressed stamped envelope and $1.

6. **American Parkinson Disease Association.** 1250 Hylan Boulevard, Staten Island, NY 10305. 1-(800)-223-APDA.

7. **American Self-Help Clearinghouse.** 75 Bloomfield Ave., Denville, NJ 07834. 1-(800)-367-6274.

8. **Ankylosing Spondylitis Association.** 511 N. LaCrenega Blvd, Suite 216, Los Angeles, CA 90048. 1-(800)-777-8189.

9. **Arthritis Foundation.** West Peachtree Street, Atlanta, GA 30309. 1-(800)-283-7800.

   Web address: http://www.arthritis.org

10. **Chronic Pain Letter.** Box 1303 Old Chelsea Station, New York, NY 10011. An excellent bimonthly newsletter that provides current informationonthe management of chronic pain to the sufferer and the professional.

11. **Chronic Syndrome Support Association.** One School Street, Suite 403, Arlington, MA 02174. 1-(781)-646-6174. Information and support about all types of chronic dieases, including TMJ and fibromyalgia. Newsletter *The Syndrome Sentinel.*

    Web address: http://www.shore.net/~cssa

12. **Fibromyalgia Alliance of America.** P.O. Box 21990, Columbus, OH 43221. 1-(614)-457-4222. National newsletter, *Fibromyalgia Times*, contains articles by health professionals on chornic pain, treatment, psychological issues, national research, government issues and questions and answers.

13. **Fibromyalgia Association of Greater Washington.** 13203 Valley Drive, Woodbridge, VA 22191. 1-(703)-790-2324. Excellent information and support concerning fibromyalgia. Subscribe to the newsletter, *Fibromyalgia Frontiers.*

    Web address: http://www.fmagw.org

14. **Lupus Foundation of America.** 4 Research Pl, Suite 180, Rockville, MD 20850-3226. 1-(800)-558-0121.

15. **Meniere's Network, Ear Foundation.** 2000 Church Street, P.O. Box 111, Nashville, TN 37236. 1-(800)-545-HEAR.

16. **MyoData/TMJ & Stress Center.** P.O. Box 803394, Dallas, TX 75380. 1-(800)-533-5121. Their newsletter, *TMJ News 'n Views,* is designed to "offer education, support and hope."

17. **National Chronic Pain Outreach Association.** 7979 Old Georgetown Road, Suite 100, Bethesda, MD 20814. 1-(301)-652-4948. Information clearinghouse. Can provide a "Support Group Starter Kit" for the formationof a local chronic-pain support group.

18. **National Commission for the Certificationof Acupuncturists.** 1424 16th St. NW, Suite 501, Washington, DC 20036. (202) 232-1404. Can provide referrals.

19. **National Fibromyalgia Research Association.** P.O. Box 500, Salem, OR 97302.

    Web address: http://www.teleport.com/~nfra

20. **National Organization for Rare Disorders.** P.O. Box 8923, New Fairfield, CT 06812. 1-(800)-999-NORD.

21. **National Self-Help Clearinghouse.** Graduate School and University Center of the City University of New York, 25 West Forty-third Street, Room 620, New York, NY 10036. 1-(212)-642-2944.

22. **Panic Disorder Education Program.** National Institute of Mental Health, National Institutes of Health, 5600 Fishers Lane, Room 7-99, Rockville, MD 20857. 1-(800)-64-PANIC.

23. **Parkinson's Educational Program/USA.** 3900 Birch Street, No. 105, Newport Beach, CA 92660. 1-(800)-344-7872.

24. **Scleroderma, fibromyalgia, and lupus** help and encouragement on the Internet.

    Web address: http://ps.superb.net/smessick/survive

25. **Scleroderma Foundation.** 89 Newbury Street, Suite 201, Danvers, MA 01923. 1-(978)-750-4499; 1-(800)-722-HOPE.

    Web address: http://www.scleroderma.org

26. **Scleroderma Research Foundation.** Pueblo Medical Commons, 2320 Bath STreet, Suite 307, Santa Barbara, CA 93105. 1-(800) 441-CURE.

    Web address: http://www.srfcure.org

27. **Spondylitis Association of America,** P.O. Box 5872, Sherman Oaks, CA 91413. 1-(800)-777-8189.

28. **TMJ Association, Ltd.** 6418 W. Washington Boulevard, Milwaukee, WI 53213. Sponsors the newsletter, *The TMJ Report.*

29. **Trigeminal Neuralgia Association.** P.O. Box 340, Barnegat Light, NJ 08006. Education, support and publications about trigeminal neuralgia.

    Web address: http://neurosurgery.mgh.harvard.edu/tna

30. **The USA Fibromyalgia Association.** Box 1483, Dublin, OH 43017. 1-(614)-851-9177. Quarterly newsletter and information about scientific findings about fibromyalgia. Information concerning support groups.

    Web address: http://www.w2.com/fibro1.html

31. **Usenet TMJ Newsgroup** on the Internet

Web address: http://www.dejanews.com

Appendix B

Bibliography

Allen, J.D., Rivera-Morales, W.C. and Zwemer, J.D. Occurrence of temporomandibular disorder symptoms in young adults with and without bruxism. *Journal of Craniomandibular Practice* 1990; 8:312-318.

Balch, J. and Balch, P. *Prescription for Nutritional Healing*, 2nd ed. Golden City Park, NY: Avery Publishing Group, 1997.

Becker, D. *Drug Therapy in Dentistry*. Plymouth: Hayden-McNer Publishing, 1996.

Boyd J.P. Prevention of migraine pain by exploiting a nociceptive trigeminal reflex: a clinical observation. Unpublished study.

Brena, S.F. (ed). *Chronic Pain: America's Hidden Epidemic*. New York: Atheneum, 1978.

Clark G.T., Beemsterboer P.L., Solberg W.K. and Rugh J.D. Nocturnal electromyographic evaluation of myofascial pain dysfunction in patients undergoing occlusal splint therapy. *Journal of the American Dental Association* 1979; 99:607-611.

Correll R.W. and Wescott W.B. Eagle's syndrome diagnosed after history of headache, dysphasia, otalgia, and limited neck movement. *Journal of the American Dental Association* 1982; 104:491-492.

Ernest, E.A., Kayne, B., Montgomery, E.W., Shankland, W.E. and Spiegel, E.A. Three disorders that frequently cause temporomandibular joint pain: internal derangement, temporal tendinitis and Ernest syndrome. *Journal Neurologic Orthopaedic Medicine & Surgery* 1986; 7:189-192.

Ernest, E.A., Martinez, M.E., Rydzewski, D.B. and Salter, E.G. Photomicrographic evidence of temporal tendinitis. *Journal Prosthetic Dentistry* 1991; 65:127-130.

Francis, J.H. *Acute and Chronic Headaches*. Irving: Aardvark, 1992.

Gelb, H. (ed). *Clinical Management of Head, Neck and TMJ Pain and Dysfunction*, 2nd ed. Philadelphia: W.B. Saunders, 1985.

Goddard, G. *TMJ — The Jaw Connection: The Overlooked Diagnosis*. Santa Fe: Aurora Press, 1991.

Gold, M.S. *The Good News About Panic, Anxiety & Phobias*. New York: Villard Books, 1989.

Greist, J.H., Jefferson, J.W. and Marks, I.M. *Anxiety and Its Treatment*. Washington, D.C.: American Psychiatric Press, 1986.

Goldman, A.R. and McCullough, V. *TMJ Syndrome: The Overlooked Diagnosis*. New York: Simon & Schuster, 1987.

Haers, P.E. and Sailer, H.F. Mandibular resorption due to systemic sclerosis. Case report of surgical correction of a secondary open bite deformity. *International Journal of Oral and Maxillofacial Surgery* 1995; 24:261-267.

Hamada T., Kotani H., Kawazoe Y. and Yamada S. Effect of occlusal splints on the EMG activity of masseter and temporal muscles in bruxism with clinical symptoms. *Journal Oral Rehabilitation* 1982; 9:119-123.

Hay K.M. The treatment of pain trigger areas in migraine. *Journal of the College of General Practice* 1976; 26:372-376.

Hendler, N.H. *How To Cope With Chronic Pain*. Boca Raton: Cool Hand Communications, 1993.

Hendler, N.H. and Alsofrom-Fenton, J. *Coping with Chronic Pain*. New York: Clarkson Potter Pub., 1979.

Jensen K. Experimental tooth clenching in common migraine. *Cephalgia* 1985; 5:245-251.

Jones C.M. Chronic headache and nocturnal bruxism in a 5-year-old child treated with an occlusal splint. *International Journal of Paediatric Dentistry* 1993; 3:95-97.

Kaplan, A.S. and Williams, G. *The TMJ Book*. New York: Pharos, 1988.

Kastan, M. Antioxidants enhance cancer drugs. *Nature Medicine* 1997; 3:1233-1241.

Lapeer G.L. Reduction of the painful sequelae of migraine headache by use of the occlusal diagnostic splint: an hypothesis. *Journal of Craniomandibular Practice* 1988; 6:82-86.

Magnusson T. and Carlsson G.E. Recurrent headaches in relation to temporomandibular joint pain-dysfunction. *Acta Odontologica Scandinavica* 1978; 36:333-335.

Magnusson T. Prevalence of recurrent headache and mandibular dysfunction in patients with unsatisfactory complete dentures. *Community Dentistry and Oral Epidemiology* 1980; 8:159-164.

Molina, O.F., dos Santos, J., Nelson, S.J. and Grossmand E. Modalities of headaches and bruxism among patients with cranio-mandibular disorder. *Journal of Craniomandib Practice* 1997; 15:314-325.

Moss R.A., Lombardo T.W., Hodgson J.M. and O'Carroll K. Oral habits in common between tension headache and non-headache populations. *Journal of Oral Rehabilitation* 1989; 16:71-74.

Murray, M.T. *Encyclopedia of Nutritional Supplements: The Essential Guide for Improving Your Health Naturally.* Rocklin, CA: Prima, 1996.

Oates, W.E. and Oates, C.E. *People In Pain.* Philadelphia: Westminster, 1985.

Oleson J. Some clinical features of the acute migraine attack: an analysis of 750 patients. *Headache* 1978; 18:268-271.

Pehman, T.J. Systemic and localized scleroderma in children. *Current Opinions in Rheumatology* 1996; 8:576-579.

Pellegrino, M.J. *The Fibromyalgia Survivor.* Columbus, OH: Anadem, 1995.

Ross, J. *Triumph Over Fear.* New York: Bantam Books, 1994.

Ryan, R.E., Sr and Ryan, R.E., Jr. *Headache and Head Pain.* St. Louis: C.V. Mosby Co., 1978.

Saper J.R., Silberstein S., Gordon C.D. and Hamel R.L. *Handbook of Headache Management.* Baltimore: Williams & Wilkins, 1993.

Seagrave A. and Covington F. *Free From Fears.* New York: Poseidon, 1987.

Sears B. *Mastering the Zone.* New York: Harper Collins Books, 1997.

Shankland W.E. Bite plane therapy: theory and fabrication. *Ohio Dental Journal* 1980; 50:40-44.

Shankland, W.E. Differential diagnosis of headaches. *Journal Craniomandibular Practice* 1983; 4:46-53.

Shankland, W.E. Ernest syndrome as a consequence of stylomandibular ligament injury: A study of 68 patients. *Journal Prosthetic Dentistry* 1987; 57:501-506.

Shankland, W.E. Trigeminal neuralgia: typical or atypical? *Journal Craniomandibular Practice* 1993; 11:108-112.

Shankland, W.E. Craniofacial pain disorders that mimic temporomandibular disorders. *Current Concepts in Dentistry of the Annals, Academy of Medicine, Singapore* 1995; 24:83-112.

Shankland, W.E. Osteocavitation lesions (Ratner bone cavities): frequently misdiagnosed as trigeminal neuralgia — a case report. *Journal Craniomandibular Practice* 1993; 11:232-235.

Shankland, W.E. Common causes of non-dental facial pain. *Generdl Dentistry* 1997; 45(3):246-252.

Siegel, B.S. *Love, Medicine & Miracles.* New York: Harper Row, 1986.

Starlanyl, D. and Copeland, M.E. *Fibromyalgia & Chronic Myofascial Pain Syndrome.* Oakland: New Harbinger Publications, 1996.

Steele, J.G., Lamey, P.J., Sharley, S.W. and Smith G.M. Occlusal abnormalities, pericranial muscle and joint tenderness and tooth wear in migraine patients. *Journal Oral Rehabilitation* 1991; 18:453-458.

Steen, V.D. Scleroderma and pregnancy. *Rheumatological Disorders Clinics of North America* 1997; 23:133-147.

Taddey, J., Schrader, C. and Dillon J. *TMJ: The Self-Help Program.* La Jolla: Surrey Park Press, 1990.

Tfelt-Hansen P., Lous I. and Olesen J. Prevalence and significance of muscle tenderness during migraine attacks. *Headache* 1981; 21:49-54.

Theodosakis, J. and Adderly, B. *The Arthritis Cure.* New York: St. Martin's Press, 1997.

Travell, J.G. and Simons, D.G. *Myofascial Pain and Dysfunction: The Trigger Point Manual. Volume 1: The Upper Extremities.* Baltimore: Williams & Wilkins Co., 1983.

Wall, P.D. and Jones, M. *Defeating Pain: The War Against A Silent Epidemic.* New York: Plenum Press, 1991.

Wanman A. and Agerberg G. Headache and dysfunction of the masticatory system in adolescents. *Cephalgia* 1986; 6:247-254.

Wasner, C. K. *Pills Aren't Enough: Stories for Emotional Healing in Chronic Illness.* Columbus, OH: Anadem, 1997.

Webby and Chang. *The TMJ Iatroepidemic: Unintentional Confessions of a Profession.* San Diego: Briernet, 1997.

Wilson, J.R. *Non-Chew Cookbook*, 6th ed. Glenwood Springs: Wilson Publishing Co., 1985.

Won, W.T.T. *Why Suffer In Silence?* Pittsburgh: Dorrance, 1995.

Appendix C

Soft Diet

Because of the importance of not chewing during the process of healing disorders of the jaws, we have prepared the following hints and suggestions for eating during this period. The only restriction in a soft diet is that of texture. All foods taken in such a diet must be soft enough, finely divided enough, or sufficiently liquid, to be swallowed without chewing. In other words, the teeth should not be brought together, although foods can be mashed between the tongue and the palate.

Such foods can, however, have all the interest and flavor and variation in temperature that the patient usually enjoys. Special attention should be given to maintaining adequate protein in this kind of diet since many of the soft foods that first come to mind are predominately carbohydrate.

If food is being prepared at home, the blender is a very helpful tool in extending the variety of such a diet. For example, soups such as vegetable-beef, clam chowder, chicken, or various stews can be pureed. Baby and junior canned foods can be improved and made more palatable for the adult with the addition of herbs and other seasonings. Foods must be soft and bland in texture, but not necessarily tasteless.

On the following pages are a few suggestions in various food categories, together with some sample menus, to relieve the tedium of cottage cheese and mashed potatoes.

FRUITS. Juices, fruit purees and sauces, such as apple sauce. Bananas, mashed and baked, baked apple (remove the skin), baked pear, etc. Cooked (peeled) peaches, apricots.

MILK AND MILK PRODUCTS. Soft cheeses, egg-nog. Milk can be added to cream soups and other dishes to increase their nutritive value. Low-fat yogurt blended with fruit makes an excellent and refreshing drink.

CONCENTRATES. Nutriment, Meritene, Ensure, or instant meals mixed with milk provide protein, some nutrients and minerals, and are available in several flavors. Nutriment is a complete meal in a can, and Meritene is a powder to be mixed with milk or juices. They are more nutritious than Sego or Instant Breakfast, which are substantially carbohydrates.

VEGETABLES. Juices, spinach chopped or pureed, eggplant, squash, mashed potatoes or carrots, turnips, parsnips. Scraped artichoke or artichoke bottoms. Well-cooked broccoli, mashed beets, pureed lima beans, peas or green beans.

SOUPS. Tomato, split pea, cream soups, gazpacho, and any others pureed or blended. Unflavored gelatin may be added to any soup to add nutritive value in the form of protein.

CEREALS. Cooked wheat, farina, milk toast, Cream of Wheat, oatmeal, corn meal mush.

MAIN COURSES. Fish fillets, poached or baked. Souffles. Soft meat loaf, soft pasta, skinless franks, ground meat, eggs, well-cooked chicken. Spaghetti, chili, or lasagna. Casseroles combining chopped vegetable, ground meat, noodles, cheese, etc.

SALADS. Gelatin salads with very finely chopped cooked fruits or vegetables or soft cheeses. Peeled and chopped or mashed tomatoes. Cold cooked vegetables with vinegar and oil dressing. Avocado.

DESSERT. Puddings, ice cream or sherbet, custard, stewed fruit, prune whip. Mousses, tapioca, rice pudding. Canned fruit topped with flavored yogurt. Canned fruit on frozen yogurt. Soft cereal bars.

SAMPLE MENUS

Breakfast

Orange or tomato juice

Eggs, soft boiled or scrambled with crumbled bacon

Cooked cereal with milk

Decaffeinated coffee, tea, or milk

Lunch

Bouillon or cream soup

Cottage cheese with canned pear, banana or grated pineapple

Yogurt or sour cream

Jello

Dinner: (Main course and vegetable)

Chopped vegetable

Soft spaghetti with meat sauce

Creamed spinach

Cheese souffle

Sliced avocado with lemon juice

Soft meat loaf

Apple sauce

Creamed carrots

Stewed tomatoes

Lasagna

Cooked zucchini marinated in french dressing

Fillet of sole poached or baked in wine or tomato juice

Mashed potatoes

Ordering in a Restaurant

The following items are from a restaurant menu and are listed here as an indication of the availability of a variety of foods within the restrictions of a soft diet:

Chicken or beef with noodles

Soups

Pasta, spaghetti

Ground sirloin steak

Eggs, boiled, poached or scrambled

Wheat cakes or pancakes

Avocado

Soft cooked vegetables (for example: zucchini, creamed spinach or tomatoes)

Potatoes, baked or mashed

Stewed tomatoes

Eggplant

Salmon steak or fillet of sole

Flounder

Fillet of haddock

Cottage cheese or apple sauce

Puddings, custard, Jello

Cheese cake or cream pies

Ice cream or frozen yogurt

About The Author

Dr. Wesley Shankland graduated from The Ohio State University with a Bachelor of Science Degree, majoring in biochemistry and zoology. He continued his education and graduated from The Ohio State University College of Dentistry in 1978. In 1993, he earned a Master of Science Degree in human anatomy, and in 1998 he completed his Doctorate in anatomy, both at OSU.

Recently named to "Who's Who in America," Dr. Shankland maintains a private practice in Columbus, Ohio, limited to the diagnosis and treatment of craniofacial and TMJ disorders. The author of over 50 national and international scientific publications, a manual of head and neck anatomy, and chapters in medical textbooks, Dr. Shankland is formerly the Chairman of Surgical Anatomy for the Scripps Implant Dentistry Education & Research Center in San Diego, California and formerly Chairman of Surgical Anatomy at the Midwest Implant Institute in Columbus, Ohio.

His memberships include the American Academy of Head, Neck & Facial Pain, the American Academy of Orofacial Pain, the American Headache Society, the International Headache Association, the American Equilibration Society, the American Association of Clinical Anatomists, the North American Cervicogenic Headache Society, and the American Association for the Advancement of Science. He is a Diplomat and Board Certified by the American Academy of Head, Neck & Facial Pain, the American Academy of Pain Management and the American Academy of Neurological and Orthopedic Surgery. Dr. Shankland is on the Board of Directors of the American Academy of Head and Facial Pain and the USA Fibromyalgia Association. He has taught over 130 courses and has presented over 90 lectures throughout the U.S., Canada, Mexico, and the Caribbean concerning head and neck anatomy, craniofacial pain, headache pain, pain mechanisms, and temporomandibular disorders. On the editorial boards of four scientific journals, Dr. Shankland is Associate Editor of the *Journal of Craniomandibular Practice.*

Dr. Shankland has seen countless patients from all over the U.S. and Canada and many foreign countries in Europe, Africa, and Central America for the diagnosis and treatment of TMJ and facial pain problems.

Among his many research projects, Dr. Shankland has discovered a muscle which is located behind the eye and may produce facial pain symptoms when injured (the zygomandibularis), a bursa of the tensor veli palatini muscle which, when injured, may cause throat and palatal pain, and a branch of the second division of the trigeminal nerve, none of which have previously been reported in the scientific literature.

Currently, Dr. Shankland is working on a book about headaches and a book about common health questions. In addition and for pleasure, he is a writer of fiction and has had three short stories published and is working on an anthology of short stories.

Dr. Shankland and his wife of over 25 years, Cathy, are both from Lima, Ohio. They have three children: Wesley III, David and Carrie. Dr. Shankland may be reached at:

TMJ & Facial Pain Center
5920 B Cleveland Avenue
Columbus, OH 43231-6881
1-(614)-794-0033

Visit Dr. Shankland's web sites at:

http://www.netset.com/ ~ docws
Or
http://members.aol.com/docws

Dr. Shankland's email address is: docws@netset.com

Index